Introduction to Physical Therapy

Introduction to Physical Therapy

Michael A. Pagliarulo, EdD, PT
Associate Professor
Department of Physical Therapy
Ithaca College
Ithaca, New York

with 94 illustrations

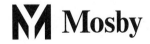

St. Louis Baltimore Boston Carlsbad Chicago Naples New York Philadelphia Portland
London Madrid Mexico City Singapore Sydney Tokyo Toronto Wiesbaden

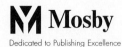
Mosby
Dedicated to Publishing Excellence

Publisher: Don Ladig
Executive Editor: Martha Sasser
Developmental Editor: Kellie F. White
Project Manager: Gayle Morris
Design and Layout: Chad Reidhead
Copyeditor: Linda K. Wendling
Manufacturing Supervisor: Betty Richmond
Cover Design: Kay Kramer

1996 EDITION

Printed in the United States of America
Composition by Wordbench

Mosby-Year Book, Inc.
11830 Westline Industrial Drive
St. Louis, Missouri 63146

International Standard Book Number: 0–8151–6714–8

95 96 97 98 99 / 9 8 7 6 5 4 3 2 1

Contributors

Barbara C. Belyea, MS, PT
Clinical Instructor
Department of Physical Therapy
Ithaca College
Ithaca, New York

Susan E. Bennett, EdD, PT
Chair, Rehabilitation Science
Director, Physical Therapy Program
D'Youville College
Buffalo, New York

Ray A. Boone, MEd, PT
Adjunct Associate Professor and Director
Department of Physical Therapy—Rochester
    Campus
Ithaca College
Ithaca, New York

Cheryl Webster Carpenter, MEd, CPTA
Academic Coordinator of Clinical Education
Department of Physical Therapy Education
University of Kansas Medical Center
Kansas City, Missouri

Jennifer E. Collins, MPA, PT
Assistant Professor
Academic Coordinator of Clinical Education
Department of Physical Therapy—Rochester
    Campus
Ithaca College
Ithaca, New York

Angela M. Easley, MPH, PT
Assistant Professor
Department of Physical Therapy—Rochester
    Campus
Ithaca College
Ithaca, New York

Clinical Instructor of Pediatrics
University of Rochester
Rochester, New York

Hilary B. Greenberger, MS, PT, OCS
Assistant Professor
Department of Physical Therapy
Ithaca College
Ithaca, New York

Michael A. Pagliarulo, EdD, PT
Associate Professor
Department of Physical Therapy
Ithaca College
Ithaca, New York

Shree Pandya, MS, PT
Assistant Professor
Department of Physical Therapy—Rochester
    Campus
Ithaca College
Ithaca, New York

Clinical Assistant Professor
Department of Neurology
University of Rochester
Rochester, New York

Dedication

This book is dedicated to my father, Anthony, for his sense of responsibility and work ethic and my mother, Louise, for her complete unselfishness and commitment to our family.

As Italian immigrants to the United States with limited educational backgrounds, they survived the hard times of the Depression and World War II through perseverance and fortitude. I am grateful to their values, sense of pride in achievement, and insistence on advanced education.

Michael A. Pagliarulo

Preface

Physical therapists (PTs) and physical therapist assistants (PTAs) are members of an exciting profession with a proud heritage. As practitioners, we focus on the health needs of the public and maintain high clinical standards, while our academic programs sustain equally high standards to prepare the graduate for patient care. Yet, too frequently, the graduates know little about the evolution of this profession, or about the interdependence of PTs and PTAs, and begin their professional education with a narrow vision of our scope of practice.

Although there exist a variety of outstanding references to address the details of the techniques of practice, there is no comprehensive text at the *introductory* level. This text fills that void. It was designed to present a broad background on the profession and practice of physical therapy for the student beginning a PT or PTA educational program. It also serves students in other health-related programs who are interested in the roles and practices of PTs and PTAs.

The organization of the text is based on a logical approach to the subjects and consists of two components: Part I (Profession) and Part II (Practice). Part I begins with a chapter on the definition and evolution of the profession to serve as a foundation. Succeeding chapters describe the scope of activities and employment settings, the physical therapist assistant, the American Physical Therapy Association, regulations to practice, and concludes with current issues. Part II provides introductory level descriptions of primary practice areas with a somewhat chronological approach. That is, the section opens with a chapter on pediatric physical therapy and continues with chapters on neurological, orthopaedic, and cardiopulmonary physical therapy; these are followed by a chapter on physical therapy for the older adult. The section concludes with a chapter on selected topics not conveniently categorized by systems or chronology.

The beginning of each chapter includes a topical outline and list of key terms to provide the reader with an orientation to the subject. References are cited throughout the text, and suggested readings are briefly described to provide resources for further study. Study questions designed to promote analysis of issues conclude each chapter.

A distinct organizational plan was incorporated into the chapters in Part II to maintain a consistent approach. This includes a general description of the practice area, common clinical conditions, evaluation principles and techniques, and treatment principles and techniques. One or more case studies in each practice area provide a context and example of the evaluation and treatment activities in the given area. In accordance with the purpose of this text, the content of Part II was comprehensive, yet introductory in nature and not intended to provide details of skills for practice.

Other factors were consistent throughout the text. These included a "people first" approach to disabilities (e.g., "individual with cardiac dysfunction" rather than "cardiac patient"), and use of female as primary gender when referring to PTs or PTAs (This is consistent with current and historical distributions.). Every attempt was made to ensure current information (e.g., policies, issues) at the time of printing; however, with a rapidly evolving profession, updates must wait for further editions.

I believe this text will serve a distinct need for a comprehensive and introductory description of the profession and practice of physical therapy. It is a result of teaching an introduction to physical therapy course for over a decade without an adequate reference resource. I look forward to comments and feedback to enhance future editions.

Michael A. Pagliarulo, EdD, PT
Ithaca, New York

Acknowledgements

This text could not have been possible without the input and support of several individuals. This begins with hundreds of students who provided constructive feedback to enhance my teaching and classroom resources. I am grateful to Dr. Charles D. Ciccone, who encouraged me to transform an idea into reality. Each contributor provided an outstanding chapter in the respective content area. Dr. Katherine L. Beissner always provided thorough and helpful consultation in her reviews of the manuscript for the chapter on Physical Therapy for the Older Adult. The photographers, Dewey Neild and Bruce Wang, were sensitive to our needs and professional in their work. Subjects in the photos (patients, family, friends, colleagues, and students) were cooperative and generous with their time. Cheryl A. Tarbell and Debby Burris, who typed the manuscripts, and Bonnie DeSombre, who constructed the graphics, somehow maintained their sanity while providing timely documents. Personnel at Mosby Year-Book, Martha Sasser and Kellie White, were encouraging and informative throughout the project. Linda and Ken Wendling at Wordbench were efficient and creative in editing the manuscript and designing the layout. Finally, I am thankful to my wife, Tricia, and children, Michael, David, and Elisa, who always expressed an interest in and support of the text. They were an inspiration not only to complete this endeavor on time, but to do so with high standards.

Michael A. Pagliarulo, EdD, PT
Ithaca, New York

Table of Contents

Introduction to Physical Therapy

Chapter 1

Physical Therapy: Definition and Development

Michael A. Pagliarulo

> "Physical therapy is knowledge. Physical therapy is clinical science. Physical therapy is the reasoned application of science to warm and needing human beings. Or it is nothing."[6]
> Helen J. Hislop, PT, FAPTA

KEY TERMS

American Physical Therapy Association (APTA)
American Physiotherapy Association (APA)
American Women's Physical Therapeutic Association
Division of Special Hospitals and Physical Reconstruction
National Foundation for Infantile Paralysis ("Foundation")
physiatrist
physical therapist
physical therapy
physiotherapists
physiotherapy
practice act
profession
reconstruction aides

The profession of **physical therapy** currently enjoys a high demand for its services and an excellent outlook for growth. Although it has become popular and received substantial publicity, confusion remains regarding its unique characteristics. For example, how does physical therapy differ from occupational or chiropractic therapy? This chapter's first purpose, then, must be to present and define this profession.

But to define it thoroughly, it is essential to also present a brief history of the development of physical therapy. A review of the past will demonstrate how the profession has responded to societal needs and gained respect as an essential component of the rehabilitation team. It will also link some current trends and practices with past events.

DEFINITION

Part of the confusion regarding the definition of physical therapy results from the variety of legal definitions which vary from state to state. Each state has the right to define this field and regulate the practice in its jurisdiction. These definitions are commonly included in legislation known as a **"Practice Act"** which pertains to the specific profession.

To limit this variety, a model definition (Box 1-1) was created by the **American Physical Therapy Association (APTA)** and was recently amended by the Board of Directors of that organization in 1993.[7]

Box 1-1

Model Definition of Physical Therapy for State Practice Acts*

Physical therapy, which is the care and services provided by or under the direction and supervision of a physical therapist, includes:

1. Examining and evaluating patients with impairments, functional limitations, and disability or other health-related conditions in order to determine a diagnosis, prognosis, and intervention; examinations include but are not limited to the following:
   - aerobic capacity or endurance
   - anthropometric characteristics
   - arousal, mentation, and cognition
   - assistive, adaptive, supportive and protective devices
   - community or work reintegration
   - cranial nerve integrity
   - environmental, home, or work barriers
   - ergonomics or body mechanics
   - gait and balance
   - integumentary integrity
   - joint integrity and mobility
   - motor function
   - muscle performance
   - neuromotor development and sensory integration

(Continued)

- orthotic requirements
- pain
- posture
- prosthetic requirements
- range of motion
- reflex integrity
- ventilation, respiration and circulation
- self care and home management
- sensory integrity

2. Alleviating impairments and functional limitations by designing, implementing, and modifying therapeutic interventions that include, but are not limited to:
   - therapeutic exercise (including aerobic conditioning)
   - functional training in self care and home management (including activities of daily living and instrumental activities of daily living)
   - functional training in community or work reintegration (including instrumental activities of daily living, work hardening, and work conditioning)
   - manual therapy techniques, including mobilization and manipulation
   - prescription, fabrication, and application of assistive, adaptive, supportive, and protective devices and equipment
   - airway clearance techniques
   - debridement and wound care
   - physical agents and mechanical modalities
   - electrotherapeutic modalities
   - patient-related instruction

3. Preventing injury, impairments, functional limitations, and disability, including the promotion and maintenance of fitness, health, and quality of life in all age populations.

4. Engaging in consultation, education, and research.

---

* From Model Definition of Physical Therapy for State Practice Acts, BOD 03-95-24-64, Alexandria, VA, 1995, American Physical Therapy Association.

This definition identifies several activities which are inherent in the practice of physical therapy. First and foremost, physical therapy begins with an evaluation to determine the nature and status of the condition. Findings from the evaluation are interpreted to establish the diagnosis, goals, and treatment plan. Treatment is then administered and modified in accordance with the patient's responses. The interventions used are physical and focus on the musculoskeletal, neurological, cardiopulmonary, and integumentary systems. Other activities which are also important for effective practice include: consultation, education, and research. Finally, it should be noted that physical therapists not only provide treatment to reduce physical disability, movement dysfunction, and pain, but also services which prevent these conditions. (See Chapter 2 for a more detailed description of the activities of a physical therapist.)

PHYSICAL THERAPY AS A PROFESSION

The model definition provides a comprehensive description of the *practice* of physical therapy. A companion document addresses the *profession* of physical therapy. This was adopted by the **House of Delegates** (policy-making body) of the APTA in 1983 (Box 1-2).[9]

Box 1-2

Philosophical Statement on Physical Therapy*

Physical therapy is a health profession whose primary purpose is the promotion of optimal human health and function through the application of scientific principles to prevent, identify, assess, correct or alleviate acute or prolonged movement dysfunctions. Physical therapy encompasses areas of specialized competence and includes the development of new principles and applications to more effectively meet existing and emerging health needs. Other professional activities that serve the purpose of physical therapy are research, education, consultation and administration.

* From Philosophical Statement on Physical Therapy (Position), HOD 06-83-03-05, Alexandria, VA, 1983, American Physical Therapy Association.

Two significant features of this Statement which embellish the model definition are that physical therapy is a profession and that it promotes optimal health and function. The latter feature—promotion of optimal health and function—is a goal established with patient/client/family input. Optimal function may meet or exceed the level prior to injury/disease or may be severely diminished as a result of impairment. The former feature of this statement—that physical therapy is a profession—warrants further discussion.

It is generally agreed that a **profession** demonstrates three characteristics: knowledge in a specific area, social value and recognized autonomy.[11] Figure 1-1 indicates that these characteristics are the most valued features of a profession.[8] It also demonstrates that a hierarchy exists with two additional traits possessing lower values. In any case, they are all important to consider.

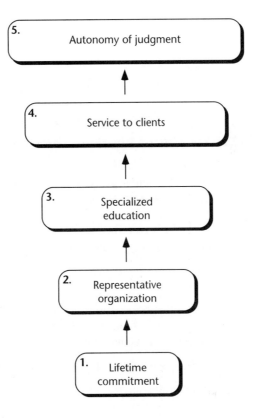

Fig. 1-1. Hierarchy of the criteria of a profession.

The first characteristic, a lifetime commitment, may seem formidable, requiring an individual's dedication to the profession. The second, a representative organization, provides standards, regulations, structure, and a vehicle for communication. In physical therapy, this is conducted by the APTA. Specialized education ensures competency to practice. For example, all licensed physical therapists must have a minimum of a four-year baccalaureate degree, and all physical therapist assistants must have an associate degree. The fourth characteristic, service to clients, is obvious in physical therapy. This provides a direct benefit to society. Finally, the last feature, autonomy of judgment, applies regardless of whether or not the therapist practices in a jurisdiction where a physician's referral is required by law. Independent and accurate judgment is inherent in every evaluation, goal, treatment plan, and discharge plan conducted by the physical therapist. This last criterion is frequently used to distinguish a professional from a technician (an individual who requires supervision).

As a profession, physical therapy emulates the criteria listed in Figure 1-1. This was not always true; therefore, the evolution of this profession included significant change and varying degrees of recognition from other professions. The next section provides a brief overview of the history of physical therapy.

HISTORICAL
DEVELOPMENT

Examining the origin and development of the profession and practice of physical therapy in the United States will serve to explain some of the current characteristics and conditions. It will also demonstrate how certain positions changed over time. The reader is referred to resources at the end of this chapter for more detailed historical accounts.

Origins of Physical Therapy

Granger described how physical measures were used in ancient civilizations to relieve pain and improve functions.[4] Massage was used by the Chinese in 3000 B.C., described by Hippocrates in 460 B.C., modified by the Romans, and accepted as a scientific procedure in the early 1800s. Techniques of muscle re-education developed from this evolution. Hydrotherapy was practiced by the Greeks and Romans through the use of baths and river worship. Finally, electrotherapy developed with the introduction of electricity and electrical appliances beginning in the 1600s.

More modern techniques of physical therapy were practiced extensively in Europe before they were employed in the United States. This was particularly true in England and France. It took the outbreak of polio epidemics and World War I to bring these techniques to the United States.

Impact of World War I and Polio

It is unfortunate that the response to widespread suffering was the impetus to develop physical therapy in this country; at the same time, this demonstrates the direct humanitarian motivation which serves as its foundation. First came the epidemics of polio (poliomyelitis or infantile paralysis) in 1894, 1914, and 1916, leaving tens of thousands of children paralyzed and in need of "physical therapy." Then, at the outbreak of World War I, the Surgeon General of the United States sent a group of physicians to England and France to learn about physical therapy techniques so that those wounded in war could be better managed. As a result, the **Division of Special Hospitals and Physical Reconstruction** was created in 1917.[2] This Division was responsible for training and managing **Reconstruction Aides** (exclusively women) who would provide physical reconstruction to the persons injured in war. These women were the forerunners of the profession and practice of physical therapy in the United States (Fig. 1-2).

During this period, polio epidemics were occurring in Vermont. A statewide program, known as the "Vermont Plan," was developed to study the cause and effects of the disease. This included health care teams that conducted field visits to provide care for the children with polio.[3] These teams consisted of orthopaedic surgeons, public health nurses, **physiotherapists** (commonly known as "physicians' assistants"), bracemakers, and stenographers. Physiotherapists became involved in determining accurate measurements for muscle strength and providing therapy through exercise and massage (Figs. 1-3 and 1-4).

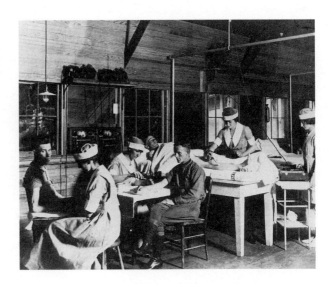

Fig. 1-2. Reconstruction Aides treat soldiers wounded in World War I at Fort Sam Houston, Texas, in 1919. (Reprinted from *Historical Photograph Packet* with permission from the American Physical Therapy Association).

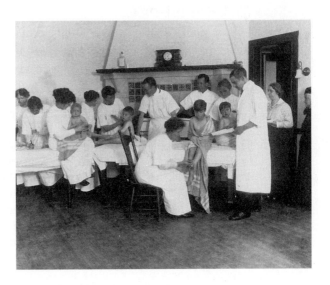

Fig. 1-3. Physical therapists and physicians work together to evaluate and treat children at a poliomyelitis clinic in New England in 1916. (Reprinted from *Historical Photograph Packet* with permission from the American Physical Therapy Association).

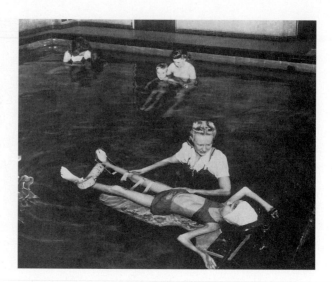

Fig. 1-4. Aquatic therapy was very effective for individuals who had polio. (Reprinted from *Historical Photograph Packet* with permission from the American Physical Therapy Association.)

Post World War I

Even when the war ended, the need for physical therapy continued. Attention shifted from preserving a fighting force to maintaining a working force. Humanitarian interests and the labor requirements of an industrial society resulted in a focus on "crippled children".[10] As the Reconstruction Aides moved into civilian facilities to address these needs, their titles and practices were plagued by confusion and ambiguity. The time had come to establish a clear identity through a national organization.

The origin of the first national organization representing *"physical therapeutics"* is traced to a meeting which was suggested by a military physician. This meeting materialized on January 15, 1921, at Keen's Chop House in New York City and was attended by 30 Reconstruction Aides and five physicians. The business included creating a national organization, the **American Women's Physical Therapeutic Association** and electing the first president, Mary McMillan.[1] The organization's first constitution indicated that it was established to maintain high standards and provide a mechanism to share information (Box 1-3).

Box 1-3

Founding Objectives of the American Women's Physical Therapeutic Association*

1. To establish and maintain a professional and scientific standard for those engaged in the profession of physical therapeutics.

2. To increase efficiency among its members by encouraging them in advanced study.

3. To disseminate information by the distribution of medical literature and articles of professional interest.

4. To make available efficiently trained women to the medical profession.

5. To sustain social fellowship and intercourse upon grounds of mutual interest.

* From Beard G: Foundations for Growth: A Review of the First Forty Years in Terms of Education, Practice, and Research, Phys Ther Rev 41 (11):843-861, 1961.

Mary McMillan was the overwhelming choice for president (Fig. 1-5). Trained in England, she is credited with becoming the first "physical therapist" in the United States.[3] As a Reconstruction Aide, she was stationed at Walter Reed General Hospital in Washington, D.C. and was appointed Head Reconstruction Aide in 1918. She also participated in the largest of seven emergency training programs for Reconstruction Aides (over 200 students) which was conducted at Reed College in Portland, Oregon.

Under the leadership of Miss McMillan, the new organization took immediate action. Two membership categories were established: charter members (Reconstruction Aides) and active members who "shall be graduates of recognized schools of **physiotherapy** or physical education, who have had training and experience in massage and therapeutic exercise, with some knowledge of either electrotherapy of hydrotherapy."[5] An official journal, the *P.T. Review,* was established and first published in 1921. Annual meetings were initiated in conjunction with annual meetings of the American Medical Association to capitalize on their programs and gain recognition. The name of the organization was changed in 1922 to the **American Physiotherapy Association (APA)**. Two males were admitted in 1923. In 1926, the journal was retitled *Physiotherapy Review.*

Two issues developed which involved physicians and took decades to resolve. The first involved identity. Physicians perceived these practitioners to be technicians or aides and suggested that this should be reflected in their title. Members of the APA believed they had a more professional status and objected to that reference. This issue was not resolved until the 1940s when physicians established physical medicine as a medical specialty. These physicians were known as **physiatrists.** The term "physical therapist" (without adding technician or aide) became acceptable thereafter.[10]

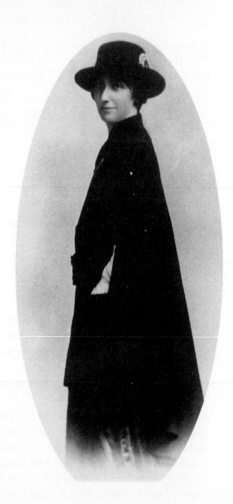

Fig. 1-5. Mary McMillan was the founding president of the American Women's Physical Therapeutic Association (precursor to American Physical Therapy Association), elected in 1921. (Reprinted from *Historical Photograph Packet* with permission from the American Physical Therapy Association.)

The second issue was more substantive and involved educational requirements. No standard educational program existed for a physiotherapist; therefore, the APA developed a suggested curriculum and published it in 1928. It was a nine-month program (1200 clock hours). Entrance requirements included graduation from a school of physical education or nursing.[1] In contrast, most of the students in the 14 training programs for the Reconstruction Aides were physical education teachers or graduates of physical education schools. A committee of the APA visited all institutions which offered educational programs for the physiotherapist and published a list of 11 approved programs in 1930.

The action by the APA did not fully resolve this issue. Greater recognition of educational programs and standards was required. The APA sought assistance from the American Medical Association (AMA) in 1933. Consequently, the Council on Medical Education and Hospitals of the AMA inspected 35 schools of physiotherapy. Based upon this inspection, as well as input from the APA and other related organizations, the AMA adopted the Essentials of an Acceptable School for Physical Therapy Technicians in 1936. Entrance requirements and length of program remained essentially unchanged; however, the curriculum was stated in detail, and other characteristics were stipulated (institutional affiliation, faculty, resources, clinical facilities). Thirteen schools were approved by the AMA in 1936.[1]

Impact of World War II and Polio

Once again national and global tragedies combined to expand the need for physical therapy and as before, the profession responded. To meet the demands of the war, eight emergency courses (six months in length) were authorized to be offered among the 15 approved full-length programs in physical therapy. These shortened courses were discontinued in 1946 when war-related demands for services dropped.

Unfortunately, the need to address individuals with polio continued. In response to repeated epidemics, the **National Foundation for Infantile Paralysis** (often referred to as the **"Foundation"**) was established in 1938 for research, education, and patient services.[2] Physical therapists continued to provide vital services for children who were affected by the disease.

The Foundation was a source of substantial support for the profession and practice of physical therapy. A past president of the APA, Catherine Worthingham, accepted the position of Director of Professional Education on the staff of the Foundation in 1944. In the same year, the first national office of the APA was established in New York City, and the first Executive Director was hired. Both of these actions were made possible by a grant from the Foundation. In that same year, a permanent headquarters and staff made it possible to create the House of Delegates to serve as the policy-making body of the organization. Other grants from the Foundation provided: (1) scholarships to recruit and retain physical therapy students and faculty; (2) funds to create a consultant to recruit and assign physical therapists for emergency work relating to polio; and (3) financial support for training in techniques fostered by Sister Kenny for individuals with polio (early application of moist heat to permit mobilization and prevent contractures).

Post World War II

The United States Army recognized the need to retain physical therapists in an organized unit to provide service to military personnel. As a result, the Women's Medical Specialist Corps was established in 1947. It consisted of physical therapists, occupational therapists, and dietitians. A physical therapist, Emma Vogel, became the first chief of the Corps and was accorded the rank of colonel.[2] Later, in 1955, the Corps became the Army Medical Specialist Corps to allow men and women to serve with commissions in the military.[1]

A major breakthrough occurred during this period in the treatment of polio with the introduction of gamma globulin and the Salk vaccine. Finally, this disease could be controlled. Physical therapists then played prominent roles during field trials of these medications, which began in 1951.

Name clarification continued as the term *physiatrist* became recognized as the title given to physicians who practiced physical medicine. **"Physical therapists"** could now practice "physical therapy"! This was reflected in the new name for the national organization, American Physical Therapy Association (APTA), in 1947 and new title for the journal, *Physical Therapy,* in 1962. This was also demonstrated in the title of the new "Essentials," which extensively revised the original document of 1936. The new title, Essentials of an Acceptable School of Physical Therapy, no longer referred to technicians. It was adopted by the AMA in 1955 and was used to approve new and existing educational programs for over 20 years. The new "Essentials" established minimum curricular standards, including a program length of 12 months.

1960s Through 1980s

This period was characterized by growth and recognition in education, practice, and research. Societal issues of this period included an aging population, health promotion, and disease prevention. Federal legislation funded health care for a variety of populations, which increased the demand for physical therapy. The profession responded with several actions.

First, policy statements were adopted by the APTA in the 1960s to clarify the preparation and use of physical therapist assistants and aides (see Chapter 3—The Physical Therapist Assistant). These positions were significant to meet the growing demands for services.

Headquarters of the APTA were relocated to Washington, D.C., in 1971 to establish stronger political involvement. Executive operations were further strengthened when the office building was purchased in Alexandria, Virginia, in 1983.

New educational programs were developed in an attempt to keep pace with the demand; curricular evolution was inherent as health care in general expanded. This period opened with an APTA policy declaring the baccalaureate degree as the minimum educational requirement for the physical therapist (1960). By the late 1970s, it became clear that a postbaccalaureate degree would be necessary to master the knowledge and skills required for competent practice. Consequently, a critical policy was adopted by the APTA in 1979 (amended in 1980) which stated that new and existing programs in physical therapy must award a postbaccalaureate degree by December 31, 1990 (see Chapter 6—Current Issues). This had a major impact on curricular development.

This period also involved an evolution of the historical link between the AMA and the APTA (formerly APA) regarding approval (accreditation) of educational programs. The APTA became more actively involved in the accreditation process. In 1974, it adopted the "Essentials of an Accredited Educational Program for the Physical Therapist," which presented a dramatic departure from the prescriptions in the 1955 "Essentials".[10] In 1977, the APTA became recognized by the United States Office of Education and Council on Postsecondary Education as an accrediting agency. "Standards for Accreditation of Physical Therapy Educational Programs" were adopted by the APTA in 1979. In 1983, after contesting the value of the AMA in the accreditation process, the APTA became the sole agency recognized to accredit physical therapy and physical therapist assistant educational programs. This recognition demonstrated the maturity of the profession.

Growth and development in the areas of practice and research resulted in new organizational units and opportunities. The American Board of Physical Therapy Specialties was created by the APTA in 1978 to provide a mechanism to receive certification and recognition as a clinical specialist in a certain area. Direct access became legal in 20 states by 1988.[10] A policy was adopted by the APTA in 1984 recognizing diagnosis in physical therapy. Regarding research, the Foundation for Physical Therapy was initiated in 1979 to promote and support research in the profession.

Several of the issues identified in this final period continue to evolve. The profession and practice of physical therapy remains responsive to societal needs. See Chapter 6—Current Issues for more description.

SUMMARY

Physical therapy is a profession which enjoys a proud heritage. From the Reconstruction Aides of World War I to the independent practitioner of today, physical therapists continue to evaluate and treat using physical means to reduce pain and improve function. This chapter provided a definition of physical therapy as a preamble to the remainder of the text. The history of the profession was traced from its origins in World War I. The influence of poliomyelitis, relationships with the AMA, development of the APTA, and recognition as a profession were described. Subsequent chapters in the text describe related aspects of the profession and practice of physical therapy.

References

1. Beard G: Foundations for growth: a review of the first forty years in terms of education, practice, and research, Phys Ther Rev 41(11):843-861, 1961.

2. Davies EJ: The beginning of "modern physiotherapy", Phys Ther 56(1):15-21, 1976.

3. Davies EJ: Infantile paralysis, Phys Ther 56(1):42-49, 1976.

4. Granger FB: The development of physiotherapy, Phys Ther 56(1):13-14, 1976.

5. Hazenhyer IM: A history of the American Physiotherapy Association, Physiotherapy Rev 26(1):3-14, 1946.

6. Hislop HJ: The not-so-impossible dream, Phys Ther 55(10):1069-1080, 1975.

7. Model definition of physical therapy, for state practice acts, BOD 03-95-24-64, Alexandria, VA, 1993, American Physical Therapy Association.

8. Moore WE: The professions: roles and rules, New York, 1970, Russell Sage Foundation.

9. Philosophical statement on physical therapy (position), HOD 06-83-03-05, Alexandria, VA, 1983, American Physical Therapy Association.

10. Pinkston D: Evolution of the practice of physical therapy in the United States. In Scully RM, Barnes ML, editors: Physical Therapy, Philadelphia, 1989, JB Lippincott Company.

11. Purtilo RB, Cassel CK: Ethical dimensions in the health profession, ed 2, Philadelphia, 1993, WB Saunders Company.

Suggested Readings

American Physical Therapy Association: Healing the generations: a history of physical therapy and the American Physical Therapy Association, Lyme, CT, 1995, Greenwich Publishing Group, Inc. A comprehensive and detailed description of the history and evolution of the profession and practice of physical therapy in the United States.

The beginning: physical therapy and the APTA, Alexandria, VA, 1979, American Physical Therapy Association. An excellent anthology of selected articles which describe the history of physical therapy and the APTA.

Hazenhyer IM: A history of the American Physical Therapy Association: 2. Formative years, 1926-1930, Physiotherapy Rev 26(2):66-74, 1946. This article describes the pertinent issues confronting the profession during this period including first published curriculum and review of educational programs, controversy over technicians vs professionals, legislation to regulate practice, and growth of the journal.

Hazenhyer IM: A history of the American Physical Therapy Association: 3. Coming of age, 1931-1938, Physiotherapy Rev 26(3):122-129, 1946. Continues description of issues in previous article as they evolved during this pre-war period.

Hazenhyer IM: A history of the American Physical Therapy Association: 4. Maturity, 1939-1946, Physiotherapy Rev 26(4):174-184, 1946. In this final article in the series, the author describes issues which involved the membership rights, Chapter organizations, further curricular changes, impact of The National Foundation for Infantile Paralysis, activities in military service, and the journal.

Matthews J: Professionalism in physical therapy. In Matthews J: Practice issues in physical therapy, Thorofore, NJ, 1989, SLACK Incorporated. This chapter is a comprehensive review of aspects which contribute to physical therapy as a profession and physical therapists as professionals.

Review Questions

1. How does the "definition" of physical therapy differ from the "philosophical statement" as defined and described respectively, by the APTA?

2. Describe the practice vs profession of physical therapy, and identify the documents that describe each.

3. Define "profession" and apply its five characteristics to physical therapy. Is it a profession?

4. How did polio and World Wars I and II affect the origin and evolution of physical therapy in the United States?

Chapter 2

Activities and Employment Settings

Michael A. Pagliarulo

" **A**ll physical therapists, regardless of title or position, function in multiple capacities, shifting from one to another as the situation demands. For example, the clinician serves as a teacher, a supervisor, a negotiator, a clinician researcher, an advocate, and a business administrator. Physical therapists in other positions not only share those functions but may assume additional ones as well."

Geneva R. Johnson, PT, FAPTA

KEY TERMS

assessment
diagnosis
direct access
evaluation
examination
forms
goals
informed consent
narrative
orthopaedics
SOAP note
treatment plan

In the past two decades, the demand for, and recognition of, physical therapists and physical therapist assistants have increased dramatically. Services have expanded in practice and employment areas where they were previously limited. This has resulted from several trends and outside influences including the aging population, federal legislation entitling children in public schools to health care, and a burgeoning public interest in personal fitness. This chapter will examine the breadth of services provided by a physical therapist and the variety of employment settings where these services exist. Recent data will be presented to describe current demographic information and employment activities and conditions.

ACTIVITIES

Direct Patient Care

The primary activity of a physical therapist is direct patient care. While physical therapists engage in many other activities, which will be described below, and in some cases no longer participate in clinical practice, patient care remains the foremost employment activity.

The entry point for an individual seeking physical therapy services is shifting from a physician's referral to **"direct access."** Burch described the preferred use of this phrase in contrast to "practice without referral," which implies no regard or interest in the critical services provided by practitioners in other disciplines.[2] Direct access, currently legal in 30 states, refers to the direct accessibility of the physical therapist to anyone seeking those services without the stipulation of a referral from another health care provider. In any case, regardless of the mode of entry, physical therapy services progress through the activities described below beginning with a thorough evaluation and terminating with discharge. (For more on direct access, see Chapter 6).

Informed Consent. An **informed consent** is required in accordance with the Standards of Practice approved by the APTA.[8] This should be obtained by the physical therapist before rendering physical therapy. The information provided to the adult (parent or legal guardian if the patient is a minor) seeking physical therapy should include: (1) a lay description of the treatment, (2) associated risks, (3) expected benefits, and (4) alternatives to recommended treatment.[6] The physical therapist should provide adequate opportunity to answer any questions the patient may have.

Initial Evaluation. This is the first critical component of the physical therapy service and must be conducted by the physical therapist regardless of the mechanism of referral. As defined in the Standards of Tests and Measurements in Physical Therapy Practice, an **evaluation** is a *judgment* based on a measurement.[9] The Standards further define **assessment** as the *measurement* (assigned value) and **examination** as the *test*. Therefore, an evaluation is a process by which physical therapists make a clinical judgment based on an assessment of an examination. It always precedes treatment. Before conducting any examinations, the physical therapist must review any available *medical records* and obtain a pertinent history through an *interview* with the individual seeking physical therapy services or a family member. The documented information is important to identify the needs of the individual/family member and cognitive status of the person seeking physical therapy.

After obtaining the medical history, the physical therapist must then select and perform the appropriate *examinations* and interpret the results. In accordance with the Evaluative Criteria for Accreditation of Education Programs for the Preparation of Physical Therapists, these examinations should include the neurological, musculoskeletal, cardiovascular, pulmonary, and integumentary systems.[3] Table 2-1 includes a list of conditions or functions identified in the Criteria which should be included in the evaluation. Figures 2-1 through 2-6 illustrate some examples of these examinations. Note that examination activities include observation, manual techniques, simple and complex equipment, and environmental assessment.

Table 2-1: Conditions/Functions to be Examined in a Physical Therapy Evaluation*

Condition/Function	Description/Example
1. Body composition	Percent body fat
2. Electrical physiological testing of muscles and nerves	Nerve conduction velocity, electromyography
3. Endurance/fitness/ conditioning	Exercise tolerance
4. Environment	Architectural barriers
5. Flexibility	Degree of soft tissue tightness
6. Functional status	Degree of independence in activities of daily living (e.g., eating, dressing, etc.)
7. Gait and balance	Degree of independence in ambulation and maintaining stable position.
8. Growth and life span development	Abilities in relation to chronological age
9. Joint integrity and mobility	Flexibility of tissues surrounding joints
10. Joint range of motion	Degree of motion available at a joint
11. Motion analysis	Use of instrumentation to measure, record, and interpret movement
12. Motor control	Neurological control of movement
13. Pain	Location, degree and type of pain
14. Perception	Interpretation of self and environment

(Continued)

Condition/Function	Description/Example
15. Physiologic response	Heart rate and blood pressure changes
16. Posture	Body/limb position
17. Pulmonary and cardiovascular functions	Status of lungs and heart especially in response to exercise
18. Reflexes	Involuntary response to stimulus; may indicate pathology
19. Righting and equilibrium reactions	Reflexes involved with maintaining balance
20. Segmental length, girth, and volume	Dimensions of limb/limb segment
21. Skin status	Presence/condition of open wounds
22. Somatosensory	Integrity of superficial and deep sensations
23. Strength	Force applied by muscles
24. Tone	Tension present in muscles

* Adapted from Commission on Accreditation in Physical Therapy Education: Self Study Report Format for Education Programs for the Preparation of Physical Therapists, Alexandria, VA, 1993 American Physical Therapy Association.

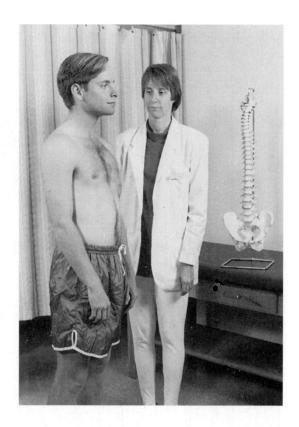

Fig. 2-1. Observation is an essential component of a physical therapy evaluation. In this case, the therapist examines the cervical posture of the patient. Compare to Figure 2-7. (Photo credit: Dewey Neild).

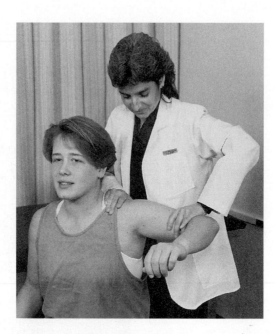

Fig. 2-2. Manual techniques such as manual muscle testing are also critical for physical examinations. In this Figure, the therapist is performing a muscle test on the patient's shoulder musculature (Photo credit: Dewey Neild).

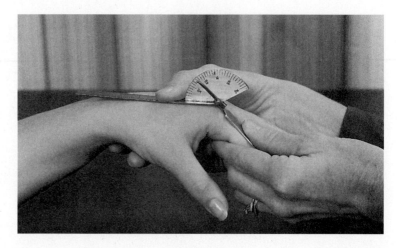

Fig. 2-3. Passive range of motion in the joints of the fingers is assessed with a simple finger goniometer (Photo credit: Dewey Neild).

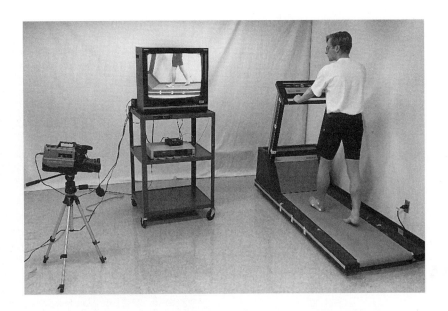

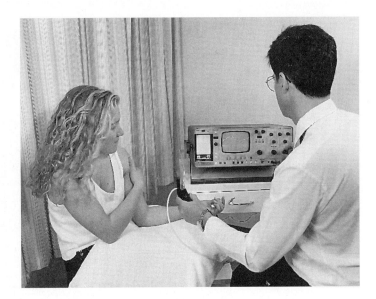

Fig. 2-4. Equipment used by physical therapists for evaluations can be complex (Photo credits: Dewey Neild). **A.** In motion analysis of the lower extremity, the patient is videotaped with markers at joint axes while walking on a treadmill. The videotape is analyzed using computer technology to provide an objective measure of performance. **B.** Electrodiagnostic equipment is used to measure the conduction velocity of nerves.

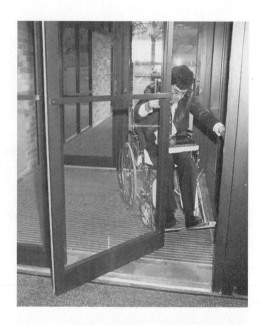

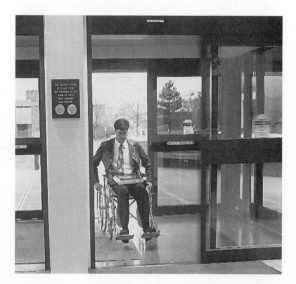

Fig. 2-5. Architectural barriers in the environment, such as doorways that are difficult to manage in a wheelchair, are also assessed by the physical therapist (Photo credits: Dewey Neild). **A.** Managing manual doorways can be difficult for individuals in wheelchairs. **B.** Automatic doorways provide excellent accessibility for individuals who use a wheelchair or assistive device.

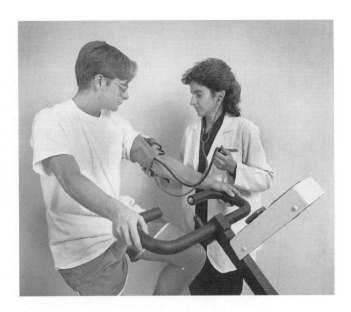

Fig. 2-6. Physical therapists can conduct cardiovascular and fitness tests using a stationary bicycle (Photo credit: Dewey Neild).

Once the examinations are completed, the findings must be interpreted to establish or confirm a **diagnosis.** The diagnosis in physical therapy is in accordance with a policy adopted by the House of Delegates of the American Physical Therapy Association (APTA) (Box 2-1).[4] This policy recognizes the professional and autonomous judgment of the physical therapist and stipulates the responsibility of referral to other practitioners when warranted.

Box 2-1

Diagnosis by Physical Therapists*

Physical therapists shall establish a diagnosis for each patient. When the patient is referred with a previously established diagnosis, the physical therapist should determine that clinical findings are consistent with that diagnosis. Prior to making a patient management decision, physical therapists shall utilize the diagnostic process in order to establish a diagnosis for the specific conditions in need of the physical therapist's attention.

A diagnosis is a label encompassing a cluster of signs and symptoms commonly associated with a disorder or syndrome or category of impairment, functional limitation, or disability. It is the decision reached as a result of the diagnostic process, which is the evaluation of information obtained from the patient examination. The purpose of the diagnosis is to guide the physical therapist in determining the most appropriate intervention strategy for each patient. In the event that the diagnostic process does not yield an identifiable cluster, disorder, syndrome, or category, intervention may be directed toward the alleviation of symptoms and remediation of impairment, functional limitation, or disability.

The diagnostic process includes the following: obtaining relevant history, performing systems review, selecting and administering specific tests and measures, and organizing and interpreting all data.

In performing the diagnostic process, physical therapists may need to obtain additional information (including diagnostic labels) from other health professionals. In addition, as the diagnostic process continues, physical therapists may identify findings that should be shared with other health professionals, including referral sources, to ensure optimal patient care. If the diagnostic process reveals findings that are outside the scope of the physical therapist's knowledge, experience, or expertise, the physical therapist should then refer the patient to an appropriate practitioner.

* From Diagnosis by Physical Therapists, HOD 06-95-12-18, Alexandria, VA, 1995, American Physical Therapy Association.

If the problem is deemed appropriate for physical therapy services, **goals** are established which are measurable, functional, and linked to the problem identified in the evaluation.[6] Input from the individual and perhaps from family members is included in establishing the goals.

A **treatment plan** is the next logical step. It is composed of selected treatment activities. It should be related to the goals and include frequency and duration.[6]

Treatment. The Criteria cited above also address treatment activities in which the physical therapist must be proficient upon graduation from a professional program. These activities are listed and described in Table 2-2. Figures 2-7 through 2-13 illustrate some examples of these treatment activities. These include manual techniques ("high-touch") and equipment ("high-tech"). At this point, the physical therapist assistant could be involved with a substantial component of the treatment as delegated by the physical therapist (see Chapter 3). Further descriptions of treatment principles and techniques are found in Part II of this text.

Re-evaluation. This is an ongoing activity and results in one or more outcomes. Depending upon the effect of the initial treatment plan, a revised plan may be established. This may include new goals. Delegated activities may be revised. The patient may be referred to another practitioner for further evaluation or treatment. The optimal result is goal achievement and discharge from physical therapy.

Table 2-2: Treatments Rendered by a Physical Therapist*

Treatment	Description/Example
1. Activities of daily living and functional training	Instruction in eating, dressing, transfers, etc., and activities to improve performance
2. Assistive/adaptive devices	Instruction in use of crutches, walkers, wheelchairs, etc.
3. Biofeedback	Sensory feedback to enhance function
4. Cardiopulmonary rehabilitation	Use of graded exercises to improve function in individuals with cardiovascular or pulmonary disease
5. Chemical agents	Use of electrical stimulation or high frequency sound waves to drive drugs through skin

(Continued)

Treatment	Description/Example
6. Cryotherapy	Therapeutic use of cold (e.g., cold packs, ice massage, etc.)
7. Developmental activities	Activities which promote progression through neurological and movement milestones
8. Electric current	Use of AC or DC current for therapeutic benefits including reduction of pain and inflammation, nerve and muscle stimulation, and wound healing
9. Electromagnetic radiations	Therapeutic use of the electromagnetic spectrum to induce deep heat (e.g., diathermy, microwave)
10. Environmental modification	Alterations in the surroundings to enhance performance (e.g., wide doorways, automatic doors)
11. Exercise	Instruction in therapeutic movement to increase strength, motion, and function
12. Gait training/balance improvement	Instruction in ambulation and stability
13. Hydrotherapy	Therapeutic use of water (e.g., whirlpool)
14. Massage	Therapeutic use of manual techniques including stroking, kneading, and stretching
15. Mechanical compression	External compression to reduce edema
16. Mobilization	Manual techniques to restore normal joint movement
17. Orthoses and external supports	Therapeutic use of braces, splints, bandages, etc., to support joints and improve function

(Continued)

Treatment	Description/Example
18. Patient/family education	Instruction to patient/family member regarding the status/treatment of the patient in regards to physical therapy
19. Posture training	Instruction in proper alignment of body segments
20. Prostheses	Instruction in use of artificial limbs
21. Pulmonary hygiene	Breathing and percussion techniques to improve pulmonary ventilation and function
22. Traction	Distraction of joints using manual or mechanical techniques

* Adapted from Commission on Accreditation in Physical Therapy Education: Self Study Report Format for Education Programs for the Preparation of Physical Therapists, Alexandria, VA, 1993 American Physical Therapy Association.

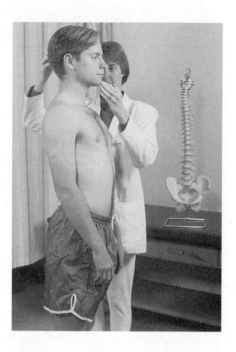

Fig. 2-7. The physical therapist corrects cervical posture with manual techniques and instruction. Compare to Figure 2-1 (Photo credit: Dewey Neild).

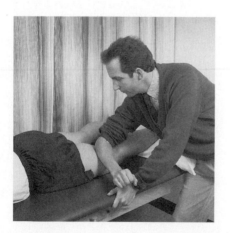 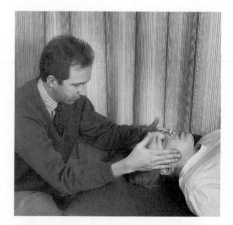

Fig. 2-8. Myofascial release techniques are effective, rigorous and gentle manual stretching techniques for soft tissue. Examples shown are in the **(A)** posterior thigh (hamstring muscle), and **(B)** temporomandibular joint region (Photo credit: Dewey Neild).

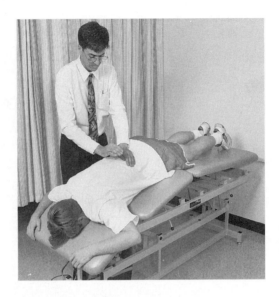

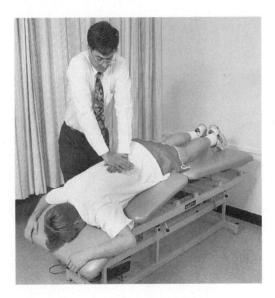

Fig. 2-9. Postural drainage involves positioning, percussion, and coughing techniques to remove fluid from specific parts of the lungs (Photo credits: Dewey Neild). **A.** A cupping technique is applied to the lower ribs in a head down position to loosen mucus in the lower lobes of the lungs (cupping done bilaterally). **B.** With outstretched arms, the therapist shakes the thoracic cage while patient exhales to encourage coughing to remove fluid from the lungs.

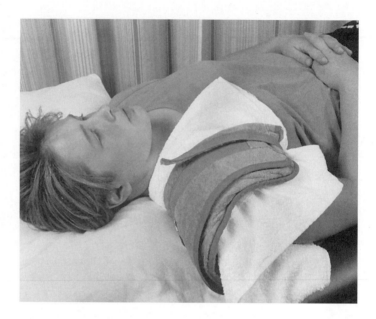

Fig. 2-10. Hot packs to the shoulder region provide an effective form of superficial heat (Photo credit: Dewey Neild).

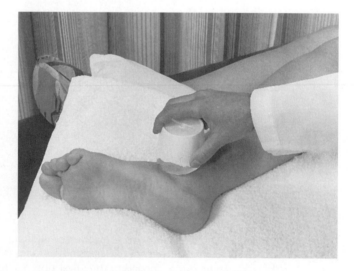

Fig. 2-11. An ice massage is administered to the ankle to decrease pain and swelling (Photo credit: Dewey Neild).

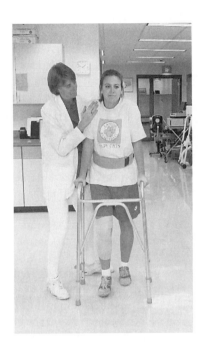

Fig. 2-12. A walker is an example of an assistive device which is used to enhance performance, such as ambulation (Photo credit: Dewey Neild).

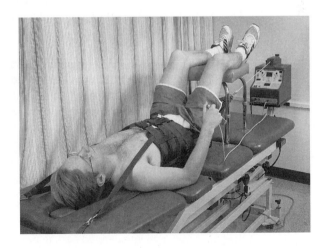

Fig. 2-13. Mechanical traction units are used to open disc spaces between vertebrae and reduce pain (Photo credit: Dewey Neild).

Communication

Written. Effective written communication is essential in the delivery of physical therapy services. Permanent records must be established to provide a baseline for future reference. They must be clear, concise, and accurate. Documentation is required by certain federal/state regulations and all insurance carriers. Fortunately, the APTA has constructed a set of Guidelines for Physical Therapy Documentation to assist physical therapists in this area.[6]

Written communication can take many formats. Documentation regarding evaluation and treatment could be written as a **narrative.** This allows maximum flexibility, but is completely unstructured. **Forms** are frequently used to provide an efficient method to record information. These are helpful, but the structure occasionally does not apply to the particular patient situation.

A third format, the **SOAP note,** combines the best attributes of the narrative and pre-established form. It is taken from the Problem-Oriented Medical Record System introduced by Weed in 1969.[10] It is structured, yet adaptable and widely used among health care practitioners. The four components are: (1) S = Subjective (what patient/family member describes), (2) O = Objective (what the physical therapist observes/measures, (3) A = Assessment (clinical judgment based upon evaluation; includes goals), and (4) P = Plan (treatment plan). The abbreviations provide an effective and efficient method to outline and document information regarding the patient.

Verbal. Verbal communication is also a significant component of the physical therapy service. The physical therapist must communicate orally with a variety of individuals including the patient, family member, referral source, and additional practitioners providing evaluation/treatment for the patient. Frequently, oral and written communication combine to provide a persuasive argument on behalf of the patient. Physical therapists must be skilled in these areas to describe their course of action.

Non-verbal. This mode of communication is occasionally overlooked as an important aspect of evaluation and treatment. It is important to note that facial expressions, body posture, and gestures often convey honest emotions (fear, pain, pleasure) which may be suppressed. In fact, Mehrabian reported that 55 percent of the impact of messages comes from the facial expression, while only 38 percent comes from the vocal component and 7 percent from the verbal.[7] Physical therapists and physical therapist assistants must always be sensitive to the non-verbal signals displayed by themselves and their patients.

Consultation

Physical therapists frequently provide consultation which is either patient centered or client centered. Patient-centered consultation refers to the service provided by the physical therapist to make recommendations concerning the current or proposed physical therapy treatment plan. It usually involves an evaluation, but not treatment.

Client-centered consultation refers to the expert opinion or advice provided by the physical therapist regarding situations which do not directly involve patient care. These consultation services are provided to clients. Examples include court testimony, architectural recommendations, academic and clinical program evaluation, and suggestions for health care policies.

Administration

Physical therapists and, to a limited extent, physical therapist assistants, may move into a variety of administrative positions. Generally, a promotion ladder exists in clinical facilities that require more administrative responsibilities at the expense of patient care activities. The individual could also shift out of the patient care environment entirely and assume an executive position within a health care or related organization. In any case, the administrative responsibilities include planning, communication, delegating, managing, directing, supervising, budgeting, and evaluating. These are particularly important when the physical therapist is owner or partner in an independent practice.

Instruction

Instruction is an inherent part of any patient care activity in physical therapy. Patients and sometimes family members are taught exercises/techniques to enhance function. This requires knowledge and skills that must be conveyed by the physical therapist or physical therapist assistant.

Instruction also occurs in the clinical facility when students are supervised during internships. Demonstration, supervision, and feedback are important to practice and perfect skills.

Physical therapists and physical therapist assistants are also involved in academic instruction. This may occur in the formal academic institution or as a continuing education program/presentation. Careers in academia are promoted by the APTA to respond to the shortage of qualified faculty in academic programs which continue to proliferate.

Research

Research in physical therapy is essential for the viability of the profession. The Foundation for Physical Therapy Research supports this activity with grants and scholarships. It has provided nearly $4 million in awards and has recently funded a Physical Therapy Clinical Research Center at the University of Iowa (see Chapter 4).

Physical therapists must continue to conduct clinical research to validate the physical therapy techniques which are used. Experimental and case studies are common research methods to answer a research question or describe a technique/outcome. These studies are neither necessarily costly nor complex and are usually generated by astute clinical observation and questioning. Consultation is available to provide assistance and guidance when necessary.

EMPLOYMENT
CHARACTERISTICS

The growth and popularity of the profession of physical therapy has created new employment opportunities. This variety and demand has had an impact on the trends and evolution regarding employment. An Active Membership Profile Survey was conducted by the APTA in 1993 to obtain current information from physical therapists.[1] Surveys were mailed to a random sample of 6000 physical therapists who were classified as active members of the APTA. There was a 49% response rate. The data from the respondents were compared to responses from previous surveys to identify trends. This section includes findings from portions of the Survey to provide a current description of employment characteristics.

Demographics

Gender. Females continue to predominate the profession of physical therapy. They comprised 74% of the respondents while males comprised 26%. This distribution has remained relatively unchanged since similar survey data were obtained in 1978. Females are also in the majority in professional level physical therapy programs, accounting for 77% of the student population.[5]

Age. The mean age of the respondents was 37.3 years. There has been a modest and progressive increase in this figure since 1978 (34.7 years); however, the members of this profession remain relatively young.

Education. A comparison of the professional degree and highest earned academic degree of the respondents is displayed in Figure 2-14. The professional degree refers to the *first* degree awarded in the area of *physical therapy*. Note that the baccalaureate degree continues to predominate. Programs which offer the postbaccalaureate degree (certificate in physical therapy) do so providing the student has at least a bachelor's degree in some field. These programs are being phased out, and this is reflected in the profiles of active member respondents who possess the postbaccalaureate certificate as their professional degree decreasing from 20.6% in 1983 to 12.2% currently. In contrast, the percent of active member respondents who possess the master's degree as their professional degree has increased from 4.5% in 1983 to 9.5% currently. This is indicative of the transition to postbaccalaureate professional education at the master's and doctoral levels.

Figure 2-14 also illustrates the highest degree attained by the respondents. This indicates pursuit of degrees beyond the professional level in physical therapy. The new degree may or may not be in physical therapy. While the baccalaureate degree continues to predominate, the figure indicates that active members are pursuing degrees at the master's and doctoral levels. Moreover, there has been a progressive increase in the percentage of the respondents who have achieved these degrees between 1983 and 1993 (18.4% to 24.4% for master's and 1.4% to 2.2% for doctoral degrees).

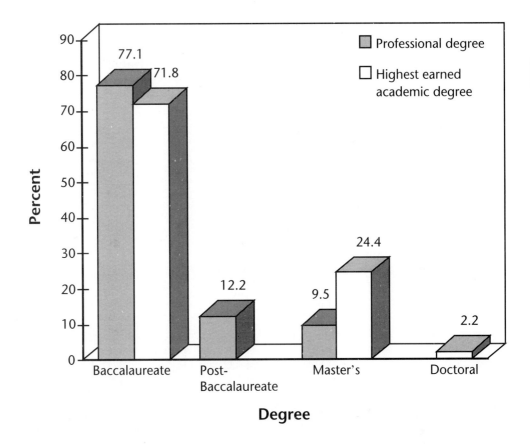

Fig. 2-14. Percent of respondents (physical therapists) to 1993 Active Membership Survey who possess the baccalaureate, postbaccalaureate, master's or doctoral degree. The Figure indicates that active members pursue higher degrees to enhance their education and careers. (Adapted from 1993 Active Membership Profile Report, Alexandria, VA, 1994, American Physical Therapy Association.)

Current Primary Position

A review of Figures 2-15A-C reveals that the majority of the respondents hold a clinical staff position in a private office with responsibilities in the area of **orthopaedics.** Other positions which provide promotion opportunities are also common (Fig. 2-15A). Regarding the facility or institution of *primary* employment, the private office has become the most common for the first time since these surveys began in 1978 (Fig. 2-15B). Most of the shift has come from the hospital setting and has contributed to the high vacancy rates there. Figure 2-15C indicates that respondents have focused their responsibilities among traditional areas of practice with an overwhelming focus in orthopaedics; however, a considerable number of respondents, 15.5%, do not practice in one area.

Other data regarding employment positions reveal that turnover remains at a substantial level. The majority of respondents, 69.8%, have been in their current position for one to five years. Although the majority of respondents hold full-time positions (63.5% salaried, 18.5% self-employed), part-time positions remain attractive (12.9% salaried, 5.1% self-employed) and support mobility.

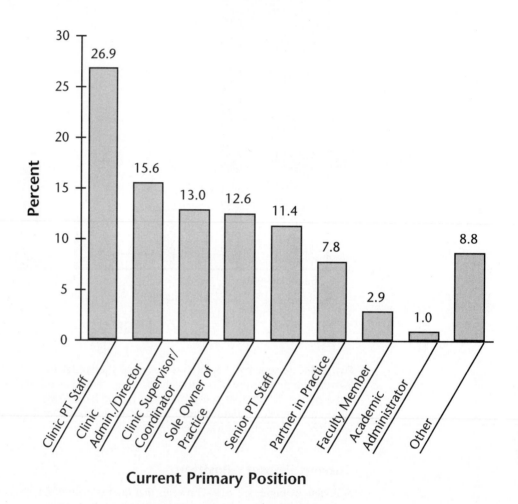

Fig. 2-15 A. Distribution of percent of respondents (physical therapists) to 1993 Active Membership Survey by current primary position. (Adapted from 1993 Active Membership Profile Report, Alexandria, VA, 1994, American Physical Therapy Association.)

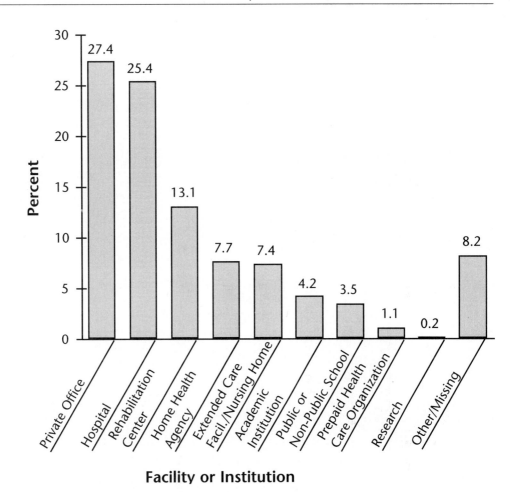

Fig. 2-15 B. Distribution of percent of respondents (physical therapists) to 1993 Active Membership Survey by facility or institution. (Adapted from 1993 Active Membership Profile Report, Alexandria, VA, 1994, American Physical Therapy Association.)

The Survey also addressed evaluation and treatment through direct access (see section on direct patient care earlier in this chapter). Over one-fourth of the respondents, 28.9%, perform direct access evaluations, and 17.9% of the respondents perform direct access treatment. These distributions have been increasing and reflect growth in the number of states which have approved legislation permitting practice under direct access for physical therapists.

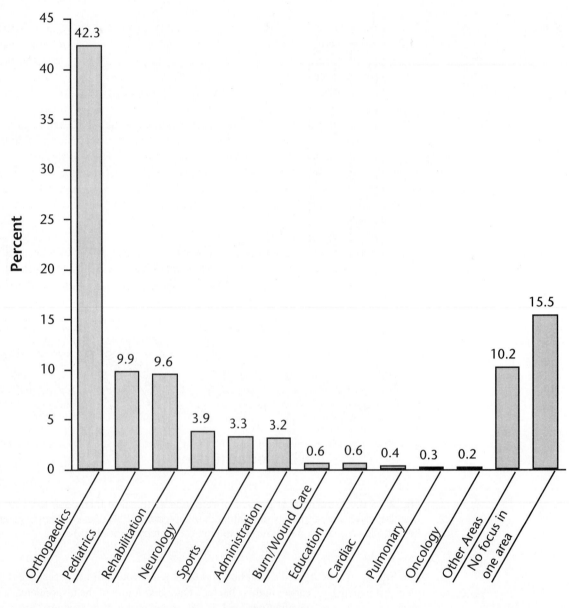

Fig. 2-15 C. Distribution of percent of respondents (physical therapists) to 1993 Active Membership Survey by area of practice. (Adapted from 1993 Active Membership Profile Report, Alexandria, VA, 1994, American Physical Therapy Association.)

SUMMARY

Although diversity and opportunity is widespread in physical therapy, direct patient care remains the primary activity of a physical therapist. This involves informed consent, evaluation, treatment, and re-evaluation. Other areas of activity include consultation, administration, instruction, and research. Regardless of the area of activity, physical therapists must communicate effectively using written, verbal, and non-verbal modes.

The majority of physical therapists are female and relatively young. The baccalaureate degree predominates as the professional degree; however, the number of therapists completing the master's or doctoral degree post-professionally is increasing. The most common employment position is that of a clinical staff member in a private office with orthopaedics as the primary area of responsibility. Turnover remains substantial, and part-time employment is common. Direct access is increasing in the areas of evaluation and treatment.

These characteristics indicate that the profession continues to thrive and evolve. Such attributes contribute to the popularity of the profession and the enthusiasm of many individuals for pursuing a career as a physical therapist or physical therapist assistant.

References

1. 1993 Active membership profile report, Alexandria, VA, 1994, American Physical Therapy Association.

2. Burch E: Direct access. In Matthews J: Practice issues in physical therapy, Thorofare, NJ, 1989, SLACK Incorporated.

3. Commission on Accreditation in Physical Therapy Education: Self-study report format for education programs for the preparation of physical therapists, Alexandria, VA, 1993, American Physical Therapy Association.

4. Diagnosis by physical therapists, HOD 06-95-12-18, Alexandria, VA, 1995, American Physical Therapy Association.

5. Goldstein MS: Professional student survey, Alexandria, VA, 1991, American Physical Therapy Association.

6. Guidelines for physical therapy documentation, Alexandria, VA, 1993, American Physical Therapy Association.

7. Mehrabian A: Silent messages, Belmont, CA, 1971, Wadsworth Publishing Co.

8. Standards of practice for physical therapy, HOD 06-91-21-25, Alexandria, VA, 1991, American Physical Therapy Association.

9. Task force on standards for measurements in physical therapy: standards for tests and measurements in physical therapy practice, Phys Ther 71(8):589-622, 1991.

10. Weed LL: Medical records, medical education and patient care, Chicago, 1970, Yearbook Medical Publishers.

Suggested Readings

Gould, JA III, editor: Orthopaedic and sports physical therapy, ed 2, St. Louis, 1990, Mosby-Year Book. A comprehensive review of evaluation and treatment techniques in orthopaedic and sports physical therapy. Arranged by technique and body region.

Hayes W: Manual for physical agents, ed 4, East Norwalk, CT, 1993, Appleton & Lange. A concise presentation on physical agents including description, purpose and effects, advantages, disadvantages, indications, contraindications, precautions, instructions, and frequency.

Hecox B, Mehretab TA, Weisberg J: Physical agents: a comprehensive text for physical therapists, East Norwalk, CT, 1994, Appleton & Lange. This text includes a thorough description of the physical agents used in physical therapy, their mechanism of action, and physiological effects.

Irwin S, Tecklin JS, editors: Cardiopulmonary physical therapy, ed 3, St. Louis, 1995, Mosby-Year Book. Presents the physiology, evaluation, and treatment of cardiac and pulmonary disorders seen by physical therapists.

Minor MA, Minor SD: Patient care skills, ed 3, East Norwalk, CT, 1995, Appleton & Lange. This text presents a comprehensive review of patient handling techniques (e.g., transfers, ambulation, etc.). Photos and a section on the Americans with Disabilities Act supplement the text.

Purtillo R: Health professional and patient interaction, ed 4, Philadelphia, PA, 1990, WB Saunders Company. This text focuses on the psycho-social aspects of interpersonal communication between the practitioner and patient.

Scully RM, Barnes ML: Physical therapy, Philadelphia, PA, 1989, JB Lippincott Company. A comprehensive text on profession and practice of physical therapy for advanced level student or practitioner.

Umphred DA, editor: Neurological rehabilitation, ed 3, St. Louis, 1995, Mosby-Year Book. Includes the theoretical foundations, evaluation, and treatment techniques of neurological disorders seen by physical therapists.

Walter J: Physical therapy management: an integrated science, St. Louis, 1993, Mosby-Year Book. This text presents current issues and strategies relating to management in physical therapy. Chapter topics include an overview of health care systems, laws and regulations, ethics, organizational behavior, marketing, and fiscal management. Case studies are used to illustrate managerial concepts.

Review Questions

1. Why is the phrase "direct access" the preferred term over "practice without referral"?

2. You go to a physical therapist for an injury sustained while skiing. Describe what you should expect at the first meeting before treatment begins.

3. Describe steps in an initial evaluation.

4. What is included in a treatment plan?

5. Discuss how you would decide which documentation format might best suit a physical therapist's needs in any given situation. Show the advantages and disadvantages of each.

6. What is the difference between patient-centered and client-centered consultation?

Chapter 3

The Physical Therapist Assistant

Cheryl Webster Carpenter

> "What matters is not the letters that come after your name, but what you can do."
> Nancy Watts, PT, FAPTA

KEY TERMS

Affiliate Assembly
Affiliate Special Interest Group
Assembly
career ladder
licensure
physical therapist assistant (PTA)
physical therapy aide
Student Assembly

"The dilemma with which physical therapy is faced is that there are not enough physical therapists to perform the essential physical therapy services, and it is apparent from identifiable trends that there will not be enough physical therapists for this purpose in the foreseeable future. Yet the need for physical therapy services is constantly growing and will accelerate in coming years."[17]

Does this sound like the opening paragraph in a current physical therapy professional journal? Actually, it is a comment made by Catherine Worthingham as a member of a panel discussion on nonprofessional personnel in physical therapy at the 1964 Annual Conference of the American Physical Therapy Association (APTA). The shortage of physical therapy personnel identified in that address was exacerbated by the continued increased demand for services. This shortage identified the need for a new kind of health care team member—one who had knowledge in the life sciences, first aid, physical therapy techniques and most important, one who could problem solve to make patient care decisions. This void was filled by the creation of a formally educated physical therapist assistant.

DEFINITION

The **physical therapist assistant (PTA)** is defined as a health care provider who assists the physical therapist in the provision of physical therapy and has graduated from an accredited physical therapist assistant associate degree program (Box 3-1).[7] The function of a physical therapist assistant is to assist the physical therapist (PT) in the delivery of physical therapy services in compliance with federal and state regulations of the practice of physical therapy. While in all jurisdictions the PTA carries out tasks delegated by the PT, the degree of supervision and autonomy varies by state.

Box 3-1

Definition of the Physical Therapist Assistant*

The physical therapist assistant is an educated health care provider who assists the physical therapist in the provision of physical therapy. The physical therapist assistant is a graduate of a physical therapist assistant associate degree program accredited by an agency recognized by the Secretary of the United States Department of Education or the Council on Postsecondary Accreditation.

* From Direction, Delegation and Supervision in Physical Therapy Services, HOD-06-93-08-09, Alexandria, VA, 1993, American Physical Therapy Association.

ORIGIN AND HISTORY

The role of the physical therapist and the utilization of support personnel have been influenced by events which have occurred over the last few decades. The Hill-Burton Act of 1946 and the subsequent amendment in 1954, provided specific funds for the construction of nursing homes, diagnostic and treatment centers, rehabilitation facilities, and chronic disease hospitals.[9] The provision for rehabilitation facilities created a new need for physical therapy.

Changes in human resource needs resulted in a shift from the exclusive use of physical therapists to the utilization of support personnel for efficient and cost-effective delivery models of patient care. The anticipated growth of the profession prompted the 1949 APTA House of Delegates to adopt the first resolution concerning the use of nonprofessional personnel.

During the 1960s, efforts were made to ensure the continued provision of health care in response to increased demand. The number of employees in the health services industry in 1960 was 2.6 million, a 54 percent increase over 1950. In 1965, the 89th Congress enacted laws which created Medicare and Medicaid. These laws began to officially recognize the need for innovative trends in health care. It was believed that the establishment and growth of new health care programs would create a need for supportive personnel. Medicare and Medicaid identified categories of these personnel and their relationships to the primary care providers.[3]

Several agencies began to investigate the creation of supportive personnel in physical therapy. These agencies included the American Association of Junior Colleges; the U.S. Department of Labor; the U.S. Department of Health, Education and Welfare; vocational schools; proprietary agencies; physician groups; nursing homes; and state health departments.

Changes in the roles and responsibilities of supportive personnel resulted in a shift in the site of preparation from the work setting (hospital) to the educational setting (campus).[4] The APTA recognized problems regarding supportive personnel shortages and unregulated educational programs. There was concern over the development of training programs without the benefit of physical therapy leadership and input.[10] A task force was established in 1964 to investigate the role of supportive personnel to the professional physical therapist and the criteria for physical therapist assistant education programs. In 1967, the task force submitted to the APTA House of Delegates a proposal for guidelines in utilizing the physical therapist assistant.

On July 5 of that same year, following deliberations, the House of Delegates adopted a policy statement regarding the standards for physical therapist assistant education programs, essentially giving birth to the physical therapist assistant. The policy statement recommended the following: "(1) that APTA was to establish the standards for the program, which also meant an attendant process of some form of accreditation; (2) that a supervisory relationship should exist between the physical therapist and the physical therapist assistant; (3) that the functions of the assistant should be identified; (4) that mandatory licensure or registration, incorporated into existing physical therapy laws, should be encouraged; and (5) that a category of membership be established in APTA for the physical therapist assistant."[16]

A subsequent policy further defined the physical therapist assistant education program as a two-year college program located in an accredited educational institution. For approval, the educational program had to provide information to the APTA Board of Directors which evaluated the program against the standards and curriculum guidelines published by the APTA.[6] This is similar to the current accreditation process followed by existing physical therapist assistant programs. Two physical therapist assistant education programs were created in 1967. Two years later, these institutions graduated the first 15 PTAs. Growth and development of new physical therapist assistant education programs was and remains phenomenal. Figure 3-1 indicates that the number of PTA education programs now exceeds the number of PT education programs.

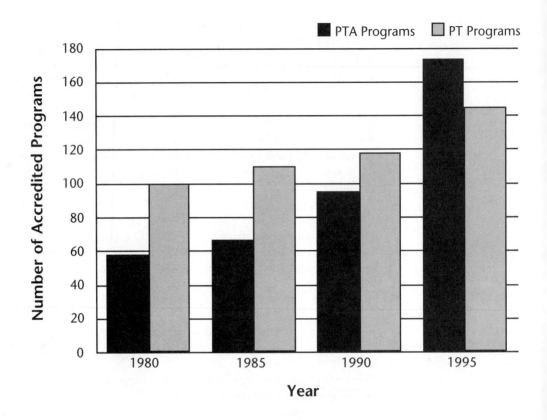

Fig. 3-1. Growth of physical therapist assistant and physical therapy education programs.

CURRICULUM AND
ACCREDITATION
STANDARDS

The curricula for all two-year associate degree PTA education programs are designed to meet the accreditation standards outlined by the **Commission on Accreditation of Physical Therapy Education (CAPTE)**. This is the same agency which accredits educational programs for the physical therapist.

In comparing the accreditation criteria for the physical therapist assistant and the physical therapist, many similarities exist. The curricula for both of these health care providers must consist of a combination of didactic and clinical learning experiences which are reflective of contemporary practice.[12,13] This is indicative of their complementary and interactive roles in clinical practice. A comparison of the similarities and differences in their educational programs provides a basis for understanding the tasks appropriate for delegation, supervision, and autonomy in clinical practice.

Educational similarities begin in their core curricula. Both physical therapist assist and physical therapy students must complete courses such as anatomy, physiology, biology, kinesiology, and general education courses that lead to the students' respective degrees awarded by the college or university. The difference in the physical therapist's education is the depth of theory provided during the mandatory advanced course work in anatomy, physiology, neuroanatomy, physics, research, pathophysiology, neurology, and pharmacology.

Courses in the professional portions of the curricula are also similar in content areas. In regard to assessment and examination techniques, specific areas must be included in accordance with accreditation criteria (Box 3-2; compare to Table 2-1).[12] Likewise, treatment techniques in specific areas must also be addressed (Box 3-3; compare to Table 2-2).[12] Figures 3-2A and B illustrate examples of a PTA performing an assessment and treatment technique.

Box 3-2

Assessment and Measurement Competencies in Physical Therapist Assistant Curriculum*

Architectural Barriers/	Pain
Environmental Modifications	Posture
Endurance	Righting and Equilibrium Reactions
Flexibility	Segmental Length, Girth and
Range of Motion	Volume
Muscle Length	Skin and Sensation
Functional Activities	Strength
Gait and Balance	Vital Signs

* From Self Study Report Format for Education Programs for the Preparation of Physical Therapist Assistant, Alexandria, VA, 1993, American Physical Therapy Association.

Clinical education is also a requirement in both curricula. Programs must provide the PTA or PT student with clinical rotations in a variety of settings and with different patient populations. Students have the opportunity to work with numerous medical diagnoses in acute care, rehabilitation, outpatient and school settings while supervised by a clinical instructor. Graduate PTAs may supervise physical therapist assistant students with additional direction provided by the Center Coordinator of Clinical Education (CCCE) or physical therapist at the facility. Graduate physical therapists serve as clinical instructors to both PTA and PT students.

Box 3-3

Treatment Technique Competencies in Physical Therapist Assistant Curriculum*

Activities of Daily Living and Functional Training
Assistive and Adaptive Devices
Balance and Gait Training
Biofeedback
Developmental Activities
Electric Current
Electromagnetic Radiation
External (mechanical) Compression
Hydrotherapy
Orthoses and Prostheses
Patient and Family Education
Postural Training and Body Mechanics
Pulmonary Hygiene Techniques
Therapeutic Exercise
Therapeutic Massage
Thermal Agents
Topical Application Including Iontophoresis
Traction
Ultrasound
Universal Precautions and Infection Control
Wound Care

* From Self Study Report Format for Education Programs for the Preparation of Physical Therapist Assistant, Alexandria, VA, 1993, American Physical Therapy Association.

Often physical therapist assistant and physical therapy students are involved in clinical affiliations at the same location. This is an opportunity for students to communicate with each other regarding the similarities in the physical therapy education programs. The delegation of tasks and the responsibility for patient follow-up could be simulated with the guidance of the respective clinical instructors.

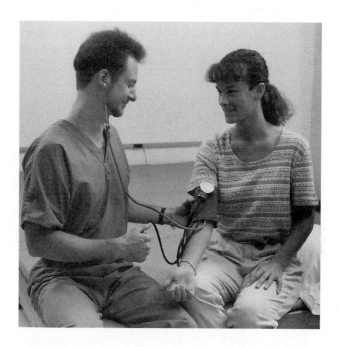

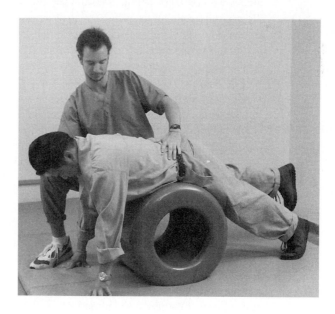

Fig. 3-2. Example of a physical therapist assistant performing: **(A)** an assessment (blood pressure measurement) and **(B)** treatment (balance and strengthening exercises).

In addition to specific content areas, the accreditation criteria emphasize that PTA program graduates practice in an ethical, legal, safe, caring, and effective manner. The graduate must understand principles of authority and responsibility, planning and time management, supervisory process, performance evaluations, policies and procedures, fiscal considerations for physical therapy, quality assurance, and be able to plan for future professional development to maintain practice consistent with acceptable standards. She/he must demonstrate the ability to modify treatment techniques as indicated in the plan of care designed by the physical therapist or acute changes in the client's physiological state. The PTA graduate must also be able to read and interpret professional literature and critically analyze new concepts.

The physical therapist assistant must also be proficient in communication. The graduate must be able to interact with patients and families in a manner which provides the desired psychosocial support; teach other health providers, patients and families to perform selected treatment procedures; participate in discharge planning and follow-up; document relevant aspects of patient treatment; and promote effective interpersonal relationships. Skill development in these areas requires knowledge and training in written, oral, and non-verbal communication.

UTILIZATION

Physical Therapist Assistant

When describing the utilization of a physical therapist assistant, it is often helpful to acknowledge and discard some of the myths that surround the topic. Utilization myths include: (1) it is essential for physical therapists to perform all physical therapy techniques with patients; (2) the assistant should only administer modalities to patients; (3) the assistant requires step-by-step instructions; (4) the physical therapist assistant is someone to whom the physical therapist delegates the noncompliant patient; and (5) the assistant is trying to take over the job of the PT. This section will dispel these myths and provide an accurate description of the roles of the PTA and PT.

While many similarities exist, differences in roles appear soon after initial employment. In a study conducted on the utilization of the PTA, Gossett reported, "Where simultaneous or near-simultaneous employment did occur, the new assistant graduate and the new physical therapy graduate appeared to function similarly, initially. The new physical therapist, however, soon was expected to accept more responsibility in the areas of departmental supervision, patient evaluations, and performance of more complex treatment procedures."[8]

The area of evaluation serves as a clear example of role distinction. It is the responsibility of the physical therapist to perform the patient's physical therapy evaluation. This requires interpreting the results of testing and using the results as a guide to set realistic goals and choose an appropriate treatment plan. This process requires understanding and judgment based on theoretical premises of life sciences which have been provided in the physical therapy curriculum.

Many aspects of the treatment plan may be delegated to the physical therapist assistant. Delegation of patient treatment after the initial evaluation requires supervision and ongoing communication. The exchange of information is crucial to physical therapy practice.

These and related responsibilities are delineated in the APTA policy titled Direction, Delegation, and Supervision in Physical Therapy Services (HOD 06-93-08-09) which states in part, "Direction and supervision are essential in the provision of quality physical therapy services. The degree of direction and supervision necessary for assuring quality physical therapy services is dependent upon many factors, including the education, experience, and responsibilities of the parties involved, as well as the organizational structure in which the physical therapy services are provided. Supervision should be readily available to the individual being supervised."[7]

The factors of education, experience, and responsibilities deserve further analysis. *Education* has been previously reviewed in the Curriculum and Accreditation Standards section. Competency in such areas as therapeutic exercise, goniometry, manual muscle testing, and modality application are requirements of a physical therapist assistant graduate.

The degree of delegation and supervision is also dependent upon *experience*. Physical therapist assistants and physical therapists continue to expand their knowledge base and skills after graduation. Continuing education courses, staff development seminars and individual inservices by colleagues take place on an on-going basis. For example, a physical therapist assistant may attend an ergonomic seating seminar. Expertise in this area may lend itself to performance of ergonomic assessments for the patient population the PTA is treating. The physical therapist may have included ergonomic instruction as a part of the treatment regimen to be performed based on patient need and, if delegated to the physical therapist assistant, the assistant's ability. If the physical therapist did not delegate this component of care to the physical therapist assistant, she/he could decide to: (1) conduct the assessment or (2) refer the patient for ergonomic assessment elsewhere.

The third factor affecting delegation is *responsibility*. Portions of the APTA policy cited above (HOD 06-93-08-09) address the responsibilities of the PT and appropriate use of the PTA for patient care activities (Boxes 3-4 and 3-5).[7] While the PT may delegate all, some, or none of the treatment tasks to the PTA, the ultimate responsibility for the physical therapy services provided to the patient including evaluations (initial, interim, and final), rests with the PT. Figure 3-3 depicts the delegation of responsibilities and interaction between the PT and PTA as a decision tree.

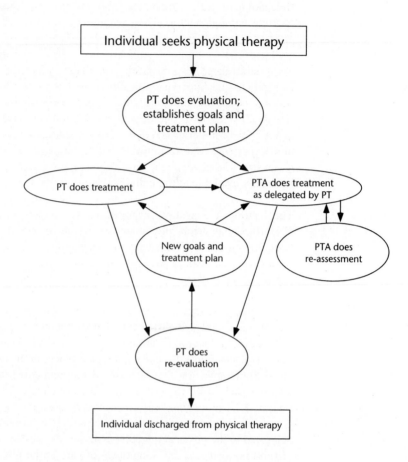

Fig. 3-3. Pathways of delegation (decision tree) involving the PT (physical therapist) and PTA (physical therapist assistant).

Box 3-4

Responsibilities of Physical Therapists Which Cannot Be Delegated to Supportive/ Paraprofessional Personnel*

Regardless of the setting in which the service is given, the following responsibilities must be borne solely by the physical therapist:

1. Interpretation of referrals when available.
2. Initial evaluation, problem identification, and diagnosis for physical therapy.
3. Development or modification of a plan of care which is based on the initial evaluation and which includes the physical therapy treatment goals.
4. Determination of which tasks require the expertise and decision-making capacity of the physical therapist, and must be personally rendered by the physical therapist, and which tasks may be delegated.
5. Delegation and instruction of the services to be rendered by the physical therapist assistant or other supportive personnel, including, but not limited to, specific treatment program, precautions, special problems, or contraindicated procedures.
6. Timely review of treatment documentation, reevaluation of the patient and the patient's treatment goals, and revision of the plan of care when indicated.
7. Establishment of the discharge plan and documentation of discharge summary/status.

*   From Direction, Delegation and Supervision in Physical Therapy Services, HOD-06-93-08-09, Alexandria, VA, 1993, American Physical Therapy Association.

Box 3-5

Utilization of the Physical Therapist Assistant*

The physical therapist of record is the person who is directly responsible for the actions of the physical therapist assistant. The physical therapist assistant may perform physical therapy procedures and related tasks that have been selected and delegated by the supervising physical therapist. Where permitted by law, the physical therapist assistant may also carry out routine operational functions, including supervision of the physical therapy aide and documentation of treatment progress. The ability of the physical therapist assistant to perform the selected and delegated tasks shall be assessed on an ongoing basis by the supervising physical therapist. The physical therapist assistant may modify a specific treatment procedure in accordance with changes in patient status within the scope of the established treatment plan.

The physical therapist assistant must work under the direction and supervision of the physical therapist in all practice settings. When the physical therapist and the physical therapist assistant are not within the same physical setting, the performance of the delegated functions by the physical therapist assistant must be consistent with safe and legal physical therapy practice and shall be predicated on the following factors: complexity and acuity of the patient's needs; proximity and accessibility to the physical therapist; supervision available in the event of emergencies or critical events; and type of setting in which the service is provided. When the physical therapist and the physical therapist assistant are not continuously within the same physical setting, greater emphasis in directing the physical therapist assistant must be placed on oral and written reporting.

When supervising the physical therapist assistant in any off-site setting, the following requirements must be observed:

1. A qualified physical therapist must be accessible by telecommunications to the physical therapist assistant at all times while the physical therapist assistant is treating patients.
2. The initial visit must be made by a qualified physical therapist for evaluation of the patient and establishment of a plan of care.
3. There must be regularly scheduled and documented conferences with the physical therapist assistant regarding patients, the frequency of which is determined by the needs of the patient and the needs of the physical therapist assistant.

(Continued)

4. In those situations in which a physical therapist assistant is involved in the care of a patient, a supervisory visit by the physical therapist will be made:
   a. Upon the physical therapist assistant's request for a reevaluation, when a change in treatment plan of care is needed, prior to any planned discharge, and in response to a change in the patient's medical status.
   b. At least once a month, or at a higher frequency when established by the physical therapist, in accordance with the needs of the patient.
   c. A supervisory visit should include:
      1. An on-site re-assessment of the patient.
      2. An on-site review of the plan of care with appropriate revision or termination.
      3. Assessment and recommendation for utilization of outside resources.

* From Direction, Delegation and Supervision in Physical Therapy Services, HOD-06-93-08-09, Alexandria, VA, 1993, American Physical Therapy Association.

Supervision is an inherent component of delegation and although certain tasks may be delegated to a PTA, as noted above, the PT remains ultimately responsible for the patient. Supervision must be provided by the physical therapist, and the physical therapist assistant should be able to request supervision as needed.

This relationship is frequently regulated by PTA:PT ratios. Although PTA:PT ratios are not defined specifically in APTA policies, these ratios may be established in a state physical therapy practice act. When establishing these ratios, the supervising physical therapist, the physical therapist assistant, and the facility management should be involved. The ratio should take into account: the *experience* of the physical therapist and physical therapist assistant, the *impairment* of the patients, the *patient caseload* per therapist/assistant, and the *accessibility* of the physical therapist by telecommunication.

For example, consider a therapist who is consulting at three clinical facilities in a rural area with one physical therapist assistant in each facility. The patient load is approximately fifteen to eighteen patients a day for each PTA. The level of impairment varies from a few patients in the intensive care units to those in the acute care sections of the facilities. In addition, the therapist needs to evaluate approximately four to five patients per day among the three facilities. The physical therapist carries a beeper and is accessible at all times. Supervision is provided in accordance with the state practice act which defines it as being available at all times through telecommunication, with weekly on-site visits.

In this scenario, the therapist is responsible for 45-54 patients of varying levels of impairment seen by the physical therapist assistants and 4-5 patient evaluations per day. As noted from this example, special consideration should be given to establish appropriate PTA/PT ratios.

Delegation in physical therapy cannot rely on myths. Facts to consider are: (1) PTAs are competent to perform many aspects of patient care inclusive of measurement and assessment techniques; (2) PTAs are competent to carry out a plan of care based on well formulated goals with general instruction from the physical therapist; (3) PTAs do not initially evaluate patients, nor do they diagnose or prognose; (4) PTAs continue to gain expertise through continuing education and work-related experience; and (5) PTAs are routinely performing the kinds of procedures that were once believed to be beyond a PTAs comprehension, just as PTs are diagnosing and performing advanced examinations once deemed to be beyond the scope of the practice of physical therapy.[2]

As the physical therapy profession progresses, the personnel within it will be required to adapt to the changes. Physical therapist assistants traditionally considered supportive personnel are now recognized as para-professionals. Although correct use of the title physical thera*pist* assistant implies that ultimate responsibility for physical thera*py* services rests with the physical therapist, partnership is a key ingredient to success in the changing environment of physical therapy.

Physical Therapy Aide

As the role and utilization of the PTA continues to evolve, confusion remains regarding the role and utilization of the **physical therapy aide**. The APTA policy which addresses the definition and utilization of the PTA similarly addresses the physical therapy aide (Box 3-6).[7] These policy statements indicate that the level of education is very limited (on-the-job training), therefore, the level of supervision is extensive. In some jurisdictions, supervision may be provided by the PTA.

The policy also indicates that in some circumstances, the title *physical therapy aide* may apply to PTA and PT students who are employed in a clinical setting exclusive of the clinical education experience. The policy makes an exception for the PTA who is enrolled in a PT program. In this case, the title PTA prevails.

Box 3-6

Definition and Utilization of the Physical Therapy Aide*

Definition

The physical therapy aide is a non-licensed worker who is specifically trained under the direction of a physical therapist. The physical therapy aide performs designated routine tasks related to the operation of a physical therapy service delegated by the physical therapist or, in accordance with the law, by a physical therapist assistant.

Utilization

The physical therapist of record is the person who is directly responsible for the actions of the physical therapy aide. The physical therapy aide provides supportive services in the physical therapy service, which may include patient-related or non-patient-related duties. When providing direct physical therapy services to patients, the physical therapy aide may function only with the continuous on-site supervision of the physical therapist or, where allowable by law and/or regulation, the physical therapist assistant. Continuous on-site supervision requires the presence of the physical therapist or physical therapist assistant in the immediate area, and the involvement of the physical therapist or physical therapist assistant in appropriate aspects of each treatment session in which a component of treatment is delegated to a physical therapy aide.

The physical therapy aide may assist patients in preparation for treatment and, as necessary, during treatment and at the conclusion of treatment, and may assemble and disassemble equipment and accessories, in accordance with the training of the physical therapy aide. The extent to which the physical therapy aide participates in operational activities, including maintenance and transportation and in patient-related activities, will be dependent upon the discretion of the physical therapist and the applicable state and federal regulations.

Students who are enrolled in physical therapist professional education programs or physical therapist assistant education programs and who are employed in a physical therapy clinical setting where such employment is not a part of the formal educational curriculum will be classified as physical therapy aides. Where their employment is part of the formal educational curriculum this policy will not apply. The physical therapist student who is a graduate of an approved physical therapist assistant program is exempt from this restriction and may be classified as a physical therapist assistant.

* From Direction, Delegation and Supervision in Physical Therapy Services, HOD-06-93-08-09, Alexandria, VA, 1993, American Physical Therapy Association.

STATE
REGULATION

Physical therapy practice is regulated in all fifty states by practice acts (See Chapter 1). These practice acts not only define physical therapy, but also the qualifications required for use of the title and practice. As an example, each physical therapist must be licensed by the state in which he or she practices. The purpose of **licensure** is to provide standards and protect the public from harm.

These acts also address the physical therapist assistant. Variations in practice acts across the United States give rise to some of the confusion regarding the utilization of the physical therapist assistant. For instance physical therapist assistants are regulated in 41 states and United States territories by licensure, registration or certification (Fig. 3-4).[15] Where these statutes exist, the physical therapist assistant is most often defined as a graduate of an accredited physical therapist assistant program. The passing score on the licensure exam is also defined by the individual state. Although some states do not regulate physical therapist assistants, supervisory requirements may be delineated in the physical therapy rules and regulations for supportive personnel. Many state regulations specify that the physical therapist may delegate aspects of physical therapy care to appropriately trained individuals. This directly affects the manner in which the physical therapist assistant is utilized and supervised.

States that do not license physical therapist assistants

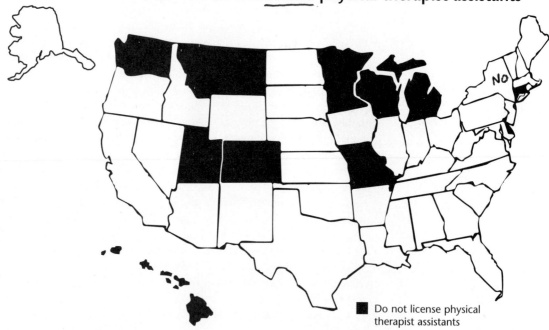

Do not license physical
therapist assistants

Fig. 3-4. States that do *not* license physical therapist assistants. (Arizona, Colorado, Connecticut, District of Columbia, Hawaii, Michigan, Minnesota, Missouri, Montana, Utah, Washington, Wisconsin. From 1994 State Licensing Reference Guide, Alexandria, VA, 1994, American Physical Therapy Association.)

These interstate variations result in a broad range of responsibilities and considerable confusion. For example, a state might mandate that the physical therapist be available at all times via telecommunication while the physical therapist assistant is providing patient care. This would allow a physical therapist to be off-site when a physical therapist assistant is treating a patient, as long as she or he is available by telecommunication. In contrast, if the practice act defines supervision as on-site, the physical therapist must be within the same facility while a physical therapist assistant is providing patient care.

The state physical therapy practice act provides the legal basis for physical therapy practice. It is imperative for the physical therapist and the physical therapist assistant to be familiar with the rules and regulations that pertain to their roles and practice in physical therapy.

EMPLOYMENT CHARACTERISTICS

Demographic characteristics and information regarding the current primary employment position of physical therapists were described in Chapter 2. These data were taken from a series of surveys conducted by the APTA. As the population of physical therapist assistants grew, it became clear that a similar PTA survey was necessary in order to establish accurate descriptive information. For this reason, the APTA conducted a survey in 1992 of the entire population of PTAs who were members of the Association. This Affiliate Membership Profile resulted in a 43.4 percent response rate (1251 survey instruments returned). The following two sub-sections are based upon data from this profile report.

Demographics

Gender. Females comprised 88.0 percent of the respondents. This degree of dominance exceeded that for the active member (physical therapist) of the APTA, which was 74 percent.[1]

Age. The mean age for the respondents was 32.9 years. This indicates a younger population than physical therapists whose mean age was 37.3 years.[1] This may be explained by the fact that the PTA position is relatively new compared to the PT position.

Education. The associate's degree was the highest earned academic degree of 83.2% of the respondents (Fig. 3-5). This reflects the degree requirement. Results also indicated that some of the respondents were pursuing a higher degree (Fig. 3-5). About half of these individuals were doing so in a physical therapy education program.[1]

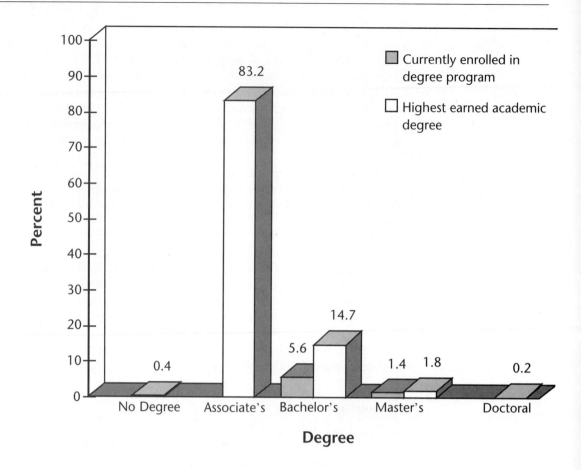

Fig. 3-5. Highest earned academic degree and enrollment patterns of physical therapist assistants. About half of these currently enrolled in a degree program were pursuing a degree in physical therapy. (Adapted from 1992 Affiliate Membership Profile Report, Alexandria, VA, 1992, American Physical Therapy Association.)

Employment Setting

In general, the percent distribution of respondents employed in a variety of settings was similar to that for physical therapists (Fig. 3-6; compare to Fig. 2-15, B). There are some notable differences, however. For PTAs, the hospital, not private office, was the primary employment setting (27.3%). On a percentage basis, over twice as many PTAs (16.4%) were employed in an extended care facility/nursing home as PTs (7.4%). This indicates the important role that PTAs perform in tasks delegated by PTs in these facilities. It also provides a context for studying the levels of responsibility of the PT and adequate supervision (see Utilization section above).[1] The current transition to a cost-containment environment may play a role in economic decisions regarding the relative staffing mix of PTAs and PTs in these settings.

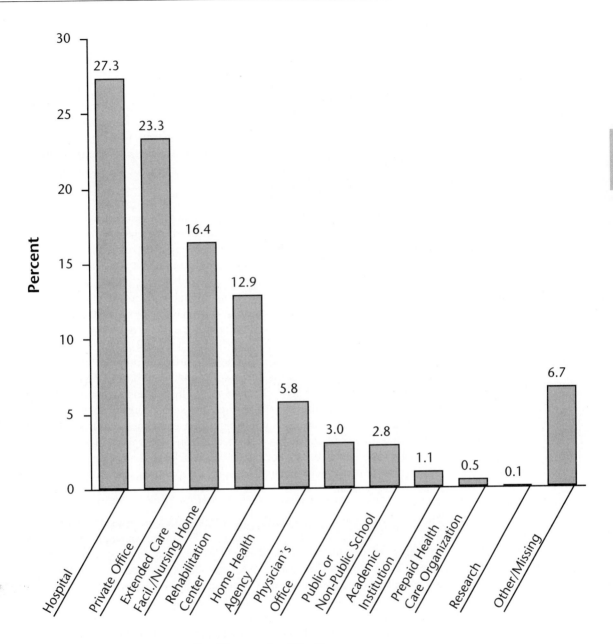

Facility or Institution

Fig. 3-6. Type of facility or institution where physical therapist assistants do all or most of their work as reported in 1992 Affiliate Membership Profile. Compare to Fig. 2-15, C for physical therapist. (Adapted from 1992 Affiliate Membership Profile Report, Alexandria, VA, 1992, American Physical Therapy Association.)

Regardless of the employment setting, the majority of respondents held full-time salaried positions (78.5%). Full-time self-employed positions were held by 5% of the respondents. Part-time employment status was also reported (13.7% for salaried positions; 1.4% for self-employed positions).[1]

Career Development

When choosing a career, students consider the field of physical therapy for a variety of reasons. The most common reason is that they want to work with patients. When considering a career as a physical therapist assistant versus a physical therapist, many factors must be taken into account. Some of these are finances, family, location of the educational program, and future career goals.

The expanding need for physical therapy personnel has resulted in an outstanding job market for the PTA. According to the United States Department of Labor projections for the year 2005, PTA is ranked the 6th fastest growing occupation among health occupations.[14] Clinical facilities compete aggressively to recruit and retain PTAs and PTs. Rural areas must provide competitive salary and benefit packages to compete with metropolitan areas because of the access to cultural activities, shopping and commerce in the urban areas. Metropolitan areas also compete with each other over salary and benefit issues. This has created a bright future for a career as a PTA or PT.

The variety of positions in physical therapy departments provides many opportunities for advancement. Like the physical therapist, a physical therapist assistant may have previous work experience in such areas as public relations, business, or education. Further analysis reveals individual characteristics such as organizational skills, in-depth knowledge of reimbursement and documentation guidelines and/or strategic planning skills. All of these can be used in a physical therapy department in a variety of capacities such as utilization coordinator, center coordinator of clinical education, or inservice coordinator. To retain valuable employees, most departments do make a concerted effort to utilize any special skills.

The issue of retention was studied by the APTA in 1988 using a survey of PTAs and PTs in hospital settings. The results revealed that PTAs remained employed at a facility for an average of five to six years, whereas PTs remained employed at a facility for an average of one to two years.[5] The PTA respondents who had resigned from acute care settings cited low salary, decreased opportunity for advancement, and a "nonflexible administration," as reasons for their decision to resign.

This prompted some facilities to begin designing **career ladders** for the physical therapist assistant similar to career ladders for the physical therapist. Eligibility requirements are based on years of experience and tenure at the facility. Duties describing the three position levels (PTA I, II, III) are categorized as clinical, administrative, teaching, educational, and professional. These career ladders are described in Table 3-1.

Table 3-1 Career Development for the Physical Therapist Assistant*

Duties	Physical Therapist Assistant Level I *(new graduate)*
Clinical Duties	Assists physical therapist in overall assessment of patier
	Assists in the implementation of patient treatment
Administrative Duties	Knowledgeable regarding department policy and procedu
	Organizes own schedule
	Carries a standard caseload
	Provides appropriate and accurate documentation
	Participates in quality improvement programs
	Participates in department administration
Teaching Duties	Teaches appropriate techniques to patients and families
	Provides inservices to staff
	Provides educational opportunities to physical therapy students
Educational Duties	Attends continuing education programs
	Attends facility meetings and orientations
	Attends departmental inservices
	Reads professional literature and remains current on physical therapy techniques
	Possesses a current CPR certification
Professional Duties	Demonstrates appropriate verbal communication skills
	Follows appropriate administrative policy
	Demonstrates professional behavior
	Actively participates in administrative meetings
	Demonstrates a willingness to participate in departmenta functions

(Continued)

Duties	Physical Therapist Assistant Level II *(2 years of experience, same job description as that of PTA I and additional duties listed below)*
Clinical Duties	Performs and interprets the results of selected measurem procedures in consultation with physical therapist
	Makes modification in patient treatment based on information for less frequent diagnoses
	Knowledgeable about community services and makes recommendations to the team
Administrative Duties	Familiar with policies and procedures and recommends changes as needed
	Cognizant of patient care priorities and facility responsibilities and adapts accordingly
	Participates on facility committees
Teaching Duties	Provides facility and community inservices
	Provides educational opportunities to physical therapist assistant students of at least one full-time affiliation per year
Educational Duties	Attends three continuing education programs per year
	Participates in one or more patient or community educational programs per year
Professional Duties	Demonstrates appropriate professional conduct
	Supportive of management response to staff

(Continued)

Duties	Physical Therapist Assistant Level III *(4 years of experience, same job description as that of PTA II and additional duties listed below)*
Clinical Duties	Able to interpret and follow the Plan of Care established by the physical therapist for less frequent diagnoses
	Assists PTA Is and PTA IIs with the interpretation of subjective and objective evaluation information
	Assesses the available community services and makes recommendations to the team
	May initiate patient care conferences after consulting wit the evaluating physical therapist
Administrative Duties	Participates in updating policies and procedures with an awareness of standards of accrediting agencies
	Provides mentoring of PTA Is and PTA IIs
	Investigates and initiates equipment repair and potential replacement
Teaching Duties	Participates in orientation of new staff
	Provides educational opportunities to physical therapist assistant students of at least two full-time affiliations per year
Educational Duties	Attends four continuing education programs per year
	Participates in APTA activities
Professional Duties	Provides insight to management regarding staff concerns

*   From Carpenter C: PTA Career Ladders, PT Magazine, 1 (1):56-61, 1993.

Another form of career development for a physical therapist assistant is a return to an educational program to pursue an advanced degree. The original policy statement regarding the physical therapist assistant supported upward mobility in education. For example, a degree in business may augment the assistant's ability to be involved in the administrative component of a physical therapy practice.

A physical therapist assistant may make the choice to pursue a degree as a physical therapist. The reasons cited are often greater autonomy, greater responsibility for patient care, and an increase in pay. If a PTA makes the choice to pursue a degree as a PT, it is especially important to note that the coursework previously completed may not be acceptable in the physical therapy program. Many physical therapy programs allow the PTA to test out of certain courses, but this is not always the case.

RIGHTS AND
PRIVILEGES IN
THE APTA

The development of physical therapist assistant education programs and the definition on the utilization of support personnel eventually led to discussion on the formation of a class of membership in the APTA for the physical therapist assistant. Heated debates over the non-professional assistant joining the APTA ensued.

In his 1969 Presidential address, Eugene Michels, PT, stated, "I am aware of the reasons given against the extension of voting privileges. Those reasons are insufficient and unconvincing. Some say that students and assistants will not know enough about the issues to vote intelligently. That argument is unsound for two reasons. First, give students and assistants half a chance, and you will soon find out what they do know. Second, every active and life member who currently holds a vote does not know what the issues are. Others fear the consequences of being out-voted by the combined power of students and assistants. If that should ever happen, and it is conceivable, the answers to the following two questions deflate that fear: (1) If it does happen, whose fault will it be? and (2) if it does happen is it necessarily bad? I find it incredible that we place so little trust in others who, we assume, are perfectly content to place their full trust in us. What a familiar ring that has!"[11]

The 1973 APTA House of Delegates approved a proposal which provided a membership category (affiliate) for physical therapist assistants. Physical therapist assistants have been affiliate members of the APTA since that action. The rights and privileges of the affiliate were different than those of the active member. The affiliate member was entitled to (1) attend all meetings, (2) speak and make motions, (3) hold committee appointments including chairman, but not any office at the national or component level, (4) serve as a chapter affiliate delegate, (5) assert a one-half vote, and (6) receive the official journal of the APTA.

In 1983, the House adopted a proposal to support the formation of an Affiliate Special Interest group to manage the concerns of the affiliate and provide more opportunities within APTA for interaction. Following this action, affiliate leaders began to formalize the **Affiliate Special Interest Group,** later known as ASIG, to identify concerns of affiliate members across the country. Regions were identified and assigned to people within the ASIG, and a chairperson was elected. This person served as the liaison with the APTA Board of Directors. The continued support of physical therapist assistants throughout the country made apparent the need for a formalized group within the APTA specifically for the PTA.

The issues surrounding categories of membership continued to plague the Association. In even numbered years, when amendments to the bylaws were proposed, topics from the past continued to be presented and defeated. The APTA Board of Directors responded by creating an organizational task force which studied the issue for two years and presented its findings to the 1989 House of Delegates.

Among the proposals was the formation of an **assembly**. The purpose of an assembly is to provide a means by which members of the same class may meet, confer, and promote the interest of the respective membership class. This proposal was adopted in 1989 along with the formation of the first assembly, called the Affiliate Assembly.

The **Affiliate Assembly** is an officially recognized component of the APTA. The officers are physical therapist assistants elected by their peers. The Assembly officers are the affiliate's formal liaisons with the APTA officers and staff. Their mission is to promote the role of the physical therapist assistant within the Association in keeping with the goals and objects of the Association.

One year after the Affiliate Assembly was created, the House of Delegates approved the **Student Assembly** (1990). The Student Assembly is comprised of physical therapy and physical therapist assistant students. This networking ability will continue to provide a forum in which PTA/PT students can better understand their roles and responsibilities in physical therapy practice.

In 1992, a motion was proposed to the House of Delegates to allow physical therapist assistants to hold office at the component level (chapter and section) with the exception of the office of president. This motion was passed in 1992 and amended in 1994 to further delineate that the physical therapist assistant was ineligible to hold an office that was in direct succession to the presidency of the component.

This motion provided additional rights and privileges to the affiliate member. The adoption of such proposals further builds on the mission of the APTA to meet the needs and interests of its membership. Over the past five years, great strides have been made for the inclusion of physical therapist assistants as affiliate members of the APTA to assume a role in the leadership of physical therapy.

FUTURE

Trends in health care will continue to influence the way in which physical therapists and physical therapist assistants are professionally prepared and function in the provision of service. Physical therapist assistant education programs will continue to expand their curricula to meet the needs of practice. The increased curriculum demands may result in a reconsideration of the degree awarded.

Continued growth in academic and clinical programs will result in greater utilization of the PTA, with an increased number hired by PTA educational programs as instructors, academic coordinators of clinical education, and program directors. Physical therapist assistants in the clinic will continue to be directly involved in the supervision of PTA students during their clinical rotations, where their advanced clinical expertise can be put to maximum use, allowing them to be positive role models.

Clinical research is another area in which physical therapist assistants will play a greater role. To a large extent, the credibility of physical therapy will depend upon continued research related to physical therapy outcome studies and provision of effective and efficient models of patient care. Such studies are continually needed to prove the worth of physical therapy services and thus ensure reimbursement for services rendered by all levels of physical therapy professionals.

The diversity of physical therapy services and society's need for these services from prevention to the provision of care for the aging population will create new demands for physical therapy practitioners. Physical therapist assistants can provide the opportunity for physical therapists to spend additional time performing patient evaluation, diagnosis, prognosis, re-evaluation, and research. This is not to say that the physical therapist assistant can replace the therapist in patient care. There will continue to be patient impairment levels that demand the presence of a physical therapist.

Physical therapist assistants will also continue to advance their skills and knowledge and become involved in departmental activities such as community education to facilitate health and wellness. Advanced clinical skills will lead to physical therapist assistant specialization and an expanded need for PTA continuing education courses.

It should be no surprise, in view of all this growth, that the APTA affiliate membership will continue to grow, relying on the Affiliate Assembly to serve as a voice of the affiliate. We should also expect to see affiliate members forming groups at the state level to address regional concerns, addressing issues of member rights and privileges at future meetings of the House of Delegates, and serving more frequently as component officers and committee chairs. Eventually, the APTA will be faced with the issue of affiliate representation on the APTA Board of Directors.

CASE STUDIES

The following case studies illustrate just two examples of the various roles the physical therapist assistant can take in the practice setting.

Physical Therapist Assistant I (Novice)

Jackie, a physical therapist working in a private practice setting, recently hired Don, a new graduate physical therapist assistant. Before assigning patients, Jackie spoke with Don regarding his course work and the physical therapy experiences he had during his clinical rotations.

Shortly after this conversation, Jackie reviews with Don the patient diagnosis, treatment plan, and precautions for a new patient with the diagnosis of a frozen shoulder (adhesive capsulitis). After the patient's third treatment, Jackie questions Don on the patient's progress. Don reports that the treatment has consisted of the exercise program Jackie had suggested but that the patient continues to have difficulty moving his arm in the correct patterns.

Jackie asks Don for suggestions of an exercise that may work better. He mentions that the patient tends to compensate with his body during pulley activities. He also adds that the corrections made to the patient's position have not worked very well. Instead, he would like to try diagonal movement patterns with verbal cueing. Jackie suggests positioning the patient supine (lying face up) and using some of the diagonal patterns with verbal and physical cueing. Don agrees that positioning the patient supine would provide better trunk stability and decrease the compensatory patterns of the trunk. Then, Jackie makes plans to work with Don and the patient during the next exercise session to problem solve together.

Physical Therapist Assistant III (Senior)

Eric, a physical therapist in a rural community hospital, has been working with the same physical therapist assistant, Cindy, for six years. After a patient evaluation, Eric confers with Cindy regarding a patient with the diagnosis of a cerebral vascular accident (stroke). He asks Cindy to review the evaluation and address any questions with him before beginning treatment in the afternoon. He requests that Cindy see the patient twice daily (BID).

Cindy reviews the evaluation and notes that the short-term goals of treatment are for the patient to sit unsupported for five minutes, and transfer three of five times with standby assistance. Eric's long-term goal is for this patient to ambulate with an appropriate assistive device (e.g., cane, walker). Cindy also notes the patient's previous history of a myocardial infarction (MI) and coronary artery disease (CAD). Cindy determines she will need to monitor blood pressure and pulse throughout the patient's treatment. The treatment sessions will be limited by the patient's endurance.

Later, Cindy walks into the patient's room where she finds him sitting in a wheelchair at bedside. She introduces herself as a physical therapist assistant on staff at the hospital.

She reminds the patient of the physical therapist who evaluated him in the morning and further explains that the physical therapist has assigned her to work with the patient on movement activities. She explains she will be taking the patient's blood pressure and pulse throughout the treatment sessions.

After informing the nurse, Cindy wheels the patient around the corner to the physical therapy gym. She transfers him to the mat, and assesses his transfer and sitting balance. She utilizes some of the neuro-developmental techniques (NDT) she learned at the fall conference to decrease the patient's sacral sitting posture. She then incorporates upper extremity activities of weight bearing and crossing the body midline. She monitors the patient's pulse and blood pressure during treatment. After she returns to the physical therapy department, she sees Eric. She tells him that the patient did well during the first session, tolerating twenty minutes of treatment before becoming tired. She provides Eric with information regarding the patient's blood pressure and pulse responses during treatment. The physical therapist concurs with the treatment approach.

After a week of treatment, the patient is able to sit unsupported for five minutes and transfers from sitting to standing with stand-by assistance. Cindy has reported this progress to Eric. After re-evaluating the patient together, they establish new short-term goals for the patient to stand with stand-by assistance for five minutes in the parallel bars, ambulate in the parallel bars for five to ten feet with minimal to moderate assistance, and perform dynamic sitting activities with extended reach, and maintain the appropriate posture three of five times without loss of balance.

The next day, Cindy speaks with the social worker and is advised that the patient has reached his insurance limit for skilled physical therapy services and will be leaving the hospital for an extended care facility. She reports this to Eric, providing him with information on the patient's functional status, manual muscle test grades, and his balance/endurance status. Eric re-evaluates the patient with the input from Cindy and develops a discharge summary including necessary equipment and plan of care for the extended care facility personnel to follow. Eric writes the final discharge note based on the patient's last physical therapy treatment while Cindy orders the necessary equipment for the patient to take with him.

SUMMARY

Many turning points exist in the growth and development of the physical therapist assistant. The APTA responded positively to an early need by creating the position of physical therapist assistant in 1967. As a result, the profession has reaped the benefits of extending its influence and thereby expanding the provision of services to more people.

As physical therapists became involved in conducting more complicated evaluations and establishing diagnoses, the utilization of the PTA was advanced to include assessment and measurement activities. Educational programs for the PTA proliferated and now exceed the number of educational programs for the PT. The American Physical Therapy Association membership responded to affiliate needs by creating the Affiliate Assembly.

Physical therapy services continue to evolve in variety and mechanism of provision. A greater understanding regarding the personnel who provide these services will result in more effective and efficient health care. This evolution will result in a profession which is empowered and prepared to face the challenges of tomorrow.

References

1. 1992 Affiliate membership profile report, Alexandria, VA, 1992, American Physical Therapy Association.

2. Bashi HL and Domholdt E: Use of support personnel for physical therapy treatment, Phys Ther 73 (7):421-429, 1993.

3. Blood H: Supportive personnel in the health-care system, Phys Ther 50(2):173-180, 1970.

4. Blood H, et al: Report of the Ad Hoc Committee to study the utilization and training of nonprofessional assistants, Phys Ther 47(11) Part 2:31-39, 1967.

5. Carpenter C: PTA career ladders, PT Magazine 1(1):56-61, 1993.

6. Collopy S, Schenck, J and Wood W: Report of a three-year study on the physical therapist assistant, Phys Ther 52(12):1300-1307, 1972.

7. Direction, delegation and supervision in Physical Therapy Services, HOD 06-93-08-09, 1993, American Physical Therapy Association.

8. Gossett R: Assistant utilization: a pilot study, Phys Ther 53(5):502-506, 1973.

9. Hill Burton state plan data: A national summary, January, 1962, United States Department of Health, Education and Welfare.

10. Hislop H: Man power versus mind power, Phys Ther 43(10):711, 1963.

11. Michels E: The 1969 Presidential Address, Phys Ther 49(11):1191-1200, 1969.

12. Self study report format for education programs for the preparation of physical therapist assistants, Alexandria, VA, 1993, American Physical Therapy Association.

13. Self study report format for education programs for the preparation of physical therapists, Alexandria, VA, 1993, American Physical Therapy Association.

14. Silverstri G: Occupational employment: wide variations in growth, Monthly Labor Review 116(11):74, 1993.

15. 1994 State licensure reference guide, Alexandria, VA, 1994, American Physical Therapy Association.

16. White B: Physical therapy assistants: implications for the future, Phys Ther 50(5):674-679, 1970.

17. Worthingham CA: Nonprofessional personnel in physical therapy, Phys Ther 45(2):112-115, 1965.

Suggested Readings

Brister S: Mosby's comprehensive physical therapist assistant board review, St. Louis, MO, 1996, Mosby-Year Book, Inc. This manual was written and "field tested" for PTA students in their second year of study who are preparing for the required board certification exam. It is designed to assist students in the review process by helping them examine their knowledge base and by pointing out areas of weakness. Includes 200 illustrations, study questions for every chapter, a comprehensive glossary, and two practice exams.

Canan B: What changes are predicted for the physical therapist assistant in the 1980s? Phys Ther 60(3):312, 1980. Guest commentary on the role of the physical therapist and the assistant as a health care team.

Carpenter C: Physical therapist assistant issues in the 1980s and 1990s. In: Matthew J: Practice issues in physical therapy current patterns and future directions, Thorofare, NJ, 1989, SLACK Incorporated. Overview of physical therapist assistant origin, education, licensure, specialization, advancement opportunities and APTA membership.

Larson CW, Davis ER: Following up the physical therapist assistant graduate: a curriculum evaluation process. Phys Ther 55(6):601-606, 1975. Survey analysis of frequency and independence in performance of 111 tasks by physical therapist assistant graduates of St. Mary's Junior College to ascertain how well they had been prepared for the demands of their jobs and discover what revisions in the program curriculum might be appropriate.

Lovelace-Chandler V, Lovelace-Chandler B: Employment of physical therapist assistants in a residential state school, Phys Ther 59(10):1243-1246, 1979. Provides an analysis of physical therapist assistant educational preparation and ethical guidelines to aid in the determination of appropriate utilization within a given facility.

Lupi-Williams F, James S and Murphy P: The PTA role and function, Clinical Management 3(3):35-40, 1983. A three part overview of the education, utilization in general practice and a job description of the physical therapist assistant in a school setting.

Robinson A, et al: Physical therapists' perceptions of the roles of the physical therapist assistant, Phys Ther 74(6):571-582, 1994. A longitudinal study which investigated physical therapists' perception of the roles of the physical therapist assistant through surveys conducted in 1986 and 1992.

Schunk C, Lippert L and Reeves B: PTA practice: in reality, Clinical Management 12(6):88-92, Nov/Dec 1992. A survey of licensed physical therapist assistants in the state of Oregon conducted by the Affiliate Affairs committee of the Oregon Physical Therapy Association, regarding how physical therapist assistants practice, supervision standards, and what PTAs believe about their utilization.

Woods: PTA twentieth anniversary, PT Magazine 1(4):34-45, 1993. Describes the evolution of the physical therapist assistant in relation to the American Physical Therapy Association and the profession.

Review Questions

1. Contrast competencies in a physical therapist assistant curriculum with those in a physical therapist curriculum.

2. Identify common myths regarding the role and utilization of physical therapist assistants. Can you combat these with "myth-breaking" facts about physical therapist assistant competence?

3. Describe the scope of physical therapist assistant competency in the practice setting.

4. What is the difference between a physical therapist assistant and a physical therapy aide?

5. Discuss the widely ranging supervision requirements for using physical therapy aides.

6. How might such skills as in-depth knowledge of reimbursement and documentation guidelines and/or strategic planning skills be used in the physical therapy setting?

7. Distinguish the roles of the following organizations: Affiliate Special Interest Group, Affiliate Assembly, Student Assembly.

Chapter 4

American Physical Therapy Association

Michael A. Pagliarulo

> "Approximately 70 percent of Americans are members of at least one association; 25 percent belong to four or more. Although the role of associations varies, these organizational entities offer forums for communication and collaboration, develop ethical standards for the individuals or groups they represent, educate members and the public, and provide a vehicle for change in society."
>
> APTA Environmental Statement

KEY TERMS

American Board of Physical Therapy Specialties (ABPTS)
American Physical Therapy Association (APTA)
annual conference
assemblies
Board of Directors (BOD)
chapter
Combined Sections Meeting
Commission on Accreditation in Physical Therapy Education (CAPTE)
districts
House of Delegates (HOD)
sections
special interest groups (SIGs)

The definition of physical therapy presented in Chapter 1 demonstrated that this field is a profession because it possesses all the qualities or criteria of a profession. One of these criteria is a representative organization. This chapter focuses on the **American Physical Therapy Association (APTA)** which is the national organization that represents physical therapy. The organization's mission, structure, and benefits are described here. We already saw a historical account of the Association in Chapter 1. Related organizations representing physical therapy interests are included at the end of this chapter.

MISSION AND GOALS

The American Physical Therapy Association is a national member-driven organization which represents the profession of physical therapy (Fig. 4-1). It is composed of more than 66,000 physical therapists, physical therapist assistants, and physical therapy students throughout the United States. Membership is strictly voluntary.

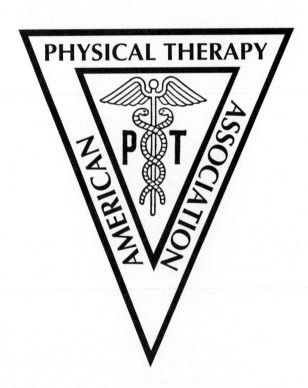

Fig. 4-1. Emblem and logo for American Physical Therapy Association. Emblem is available as pin for members only. Reprinted with permission from the American Physical Therapy Association.

In 1993, the House of Delegates of the APTA adopted a mission statement and related policy. The statement (Box 4-1)[2] and policy (Box 4-2),[6] which are shown below, demonstrate the profession's interest in serving the public and its members through practice, education, and research.

Box 4-1

Mission of the American Physical Therapy Association*

The mission of the **American Physical Therapy Association (APTA)**, the principle membership organization representing and promoting the profession of physical therapy, is to further the profession's role in the prevention, diagnosis, and treatment of movement dysfunctions and the enhancement of the physical health and functional abilities of members of the public.

---

* From APTA Mission Statement, HOD 06-93-05-05, Alexandria, VA, 1993, American Physical Therapy Association.

Box 4-2

Policy on the American Physical Therapy (APTA) Association Mission Statement*

To fulfill the American Physical Therapy Association's Mission to meet the needs and interests of its members and to promote physical therapy as a vital professional career, the Association shall:

- Promote physical therapy care and services through the establishment, maintenance, and promotion of ethical principles and quality standards for practice, education, and research;
- Influence policy in the public and private sectors;
- Enable physical therapy practitioners to improve their skills, knowledge, and operations in the interest of furthering the profession;
- Develop and improve the art and science of physical therapy, including practice, education, and research;
- Facilitate a common understanding and appreciation for the diversity of the profession, the membership, and the communities we serve; and
- Maintain a stable and diverse financial base from which to fund the programs, services, and operations that support this mission.

---

* From Policy on APTA Mission Statement, HOD 06-93-06-07, Alexandria, VA, American Physical Therapy Association, 1993.

Goals for the APTA are established annually by the Board of Directors. They are then reviewed and approved by the House of Delegates (HOD). The goals for 1996 were approved by the HOD in June 1995 and are presented in Box 4-3.[5] These goals direct the activities and funding priorities for the new year.

Box 4-3

1996 Goals that Represent the Priorities of the APTA *

GOAL I: Participate actively in shaping the current and emerging health care environment to promote the development of high-quality health care services and to further the recognition of and support for the role of physical therapy.

GOAL II: Stimulate innovation in the practice of physical therapy that supports the professional well-being of physical therapists and physical therapist assistants.

GOAL III: Increase American Physical Therapy Association's responsiveness to the needs of current and future members.

GOAL IV: Stimulate innovation in physical therapy education and professional development at all levels to ensure currency with the changing environments in health care and education and with student and professional needs.

GOAL V: Stimulate research to further the science of physical therapy, to influence current and emerging health care policies, and to advance the profession.

GOAL VI: Facilitate the development, distribution, and utilization of physical therapy human resources to provide sufficient, consistent, and high-quality services.

GOAL VII: Develop and strengthen coalitions with other professional organizations for the purpose of identifying mutually beneficial points of collaboration and advancing common goals related to the provision of services.

These goals are based on the assumption that the areas of education, research, and practice are the implicit foundation for accomplishment of the goals. The Association's awareness of cultural diversity, its commitment to expanding minority representation and participation in physical therapy, and its commitment to equal opportunity for all members permeate these goals.

* From 1996 Goals that Represent the Priorities of the Association, HOD 06-95-15-27, Alexandria, VA, 1995, American Physical Therapy Association.

ORGANIZATIONAL
STRUCTURE

The organizational structure of the APTA is depicted in Figure 4-2. This structure provides a three-tiered approach (local, state, and national) to serve the members and the public. Each level is described in this section beginning with the primary unit, the membership.

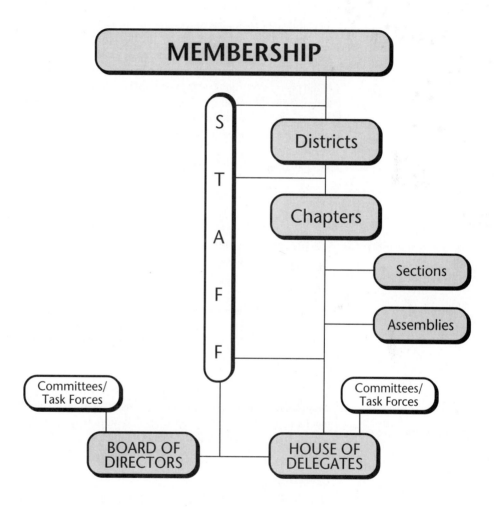

Fig. 4-2. Organizational chart of the American Physical Therapy Association. Note how the membership drives this organization. Staff members provide support at all levels including membership, districts (local), chapters (state), and House of Delegates/Board of Directors (national).

Membership

As stated above, membership in the APTA is voluntary, however, it is estimated that approximately two-thirds of licensed physical therapists in the United States are members. This provides strength and diversity to the organization.

The primary membership categories of the APTA are active (physical therapist), affiliate (physical therapist assistant), and their respective student categories, student and student affiliate. Other categories include graduate student, life (retired), honorary (not a physical therapist or physical therapist assistant), and Catherine Worthingham Fellow of the APTA (active member for at least 15 years who has made notable contributions to the profession, may use initials FAPTA). Requirements for membership include graduation from (or enrollment in) an educational program approved (or seeking candidacy) by a recognized accrediting agency. In addition, the applicant must sign a pledge indicating compliance with the Code of Ethics (active and related categories) or Standards of Ethical Conduct for the Physical Therapist Assistant (affiliate and related categories) and pay dues.

Service to the membership has always been one of the main purposes of the APTA. Likewise, members have had a sense of pride and commitment to the organization. In fact, during the formative years of the profession, membership in this organization was considered the standard for competence. This proud heritage remains today; however, membership is not required to demonstrate competence.

Districts

Figure 4-2 indicates that **districts** are the most local organizational unit in the structure of the APTA. Districts do not exist in all jurisdictions, such as small states. Membership is automatic where they do exist and may be based upon location of residence or employment as provided in the Bylaws of the APTA.

Districts are more common in locations with high population densities or large geographical areas and frequently consist of one or more counties. This provides a mechanism for convenient meetings and participation. It also provides a basis for representation in a body which conducts business at the next level of organization, the chapter.

Chapters

In accordance with the Standing Rules of the American Physical Therapy Association, a **chapter** "must coincide with or be confined within the legally constituted boundaries of a state, territory, or commonwealth of the United States or the District of Columbia."[7] In 1995, the APTA consisted of 52 chapters, one for each state, the District of Columbia, and Puerto Rico. Membership in a chapter is *automatic* and based upon location of residence, employment, education, or greatest active participation (in the last case, only in an immediately adjacent chapter). In contrast to districts which are not permitted to assess dues, each chapter requires dues for active and affiliate members, and in a few cases, student categories.

Chapters are an important component of the APTA. They provide a mechanism for participation at a state level and proportionate representation at the national level (see House of Delegates, below). Participation is facilitated through authorized special interest groups and assemblies to address the needs of recognized subsidiary groups. They also provide an important voice for members at the state level of government. This is essential to maintain statewide legislation and regulations appropriate to the profession and practice of physical therapy.

Sections

Sections are organized at the national level. In accordance with the Bylaws of the APTA, they provide an opportunity for members with similar areas of interest to "meet, confer, and promote the interests of the respective sections."[3] Membership in one or more of the 19 sections listed in Table 4-1 is voluntary. Students are also encouraged to join.

Table 4-1: Sections of the American Physical Therapy Association*

Section	Area(s) of Interest	Publication(s)
1. Acute Care/ Hospital Clinical Practice	Physical therapists practicing in acute care/hospital setting.	Acute Care Perspectives
2. Administration	Management philosophies and trends in practice.	The Resource
3. Aquatic Physical Therapy	Ideas and skills in treatment techniques in aquatic environment.	Aquatic Physical Therapy Report; Waterlines Newsletter
4. Cardiopulmonary	Heart and lung dysfunctions due to disease, injury, or birth defects.	Cardiopulmonary Physical Therapy Journal; Cardiopulmonary Record
5. Clinical Electrophysiology	Electrotherapeutic, electrodiagnostic, and electrokinesiologic procedures.	Journal of Clinical Electrophysiology; Clinical Electrophysiology
6. Community Health	Practice in home or community setting.	Quarterly Report
7. Education	Development and improvement of academic and clinical education.	Journal of Physical Therapy Education; The Bulletin
8. Geriatrics	Specific problems of older persons.	Issues on Aging

(Continued)

Section	Area(s) of Interest	Publication(s)
9. Hand Rehabilitation	Hand and upper extremity rehabilitation.	Section on Hand Rehabilitation Newsletter
10. Health Policy, Legislation, and Regulation	Health policy and legislation including licensure and related regulations.	Health Policy, Legislation, and Regulation Newsletter
11. Neurology	Developments and techniques concerning neurologic disorders.	Neurology Report; Neuro Notes
12. Oncology	Physical therapy for individuals with cancer.	Rehabilitation in Oncology
13. Orthopaedics	Examination and treatment of patients with musculoskeletal disorders.	Orthopaedic Physical Therapy Practice; Journal of Orthopaedic and Sports Physical Therapy
14. Pediatrics	Rehabilitation and disability prevention for the child.	Pediatric Physical Therapy; Section on Pediatrics Newsletter
15. Private Practice	Independent practice of physical therapy, business success, and quality care.	Physical Therapy Today
16. Research	Clinical and basic scientific research.	Section on Research Newsletter
17. Sports Physical Therapy	Management of athletic injuries.	Journal of Orthopaedic and Sports Physical Therapy; Section Newsletter
18. Veterans Affairs	High quality health care in VA medical centers.	Vantage Point
19. Women's Health	Physical and emotional health of women of all ages.	Journal of Obstetric and Gynecologic Physical Therapy

*   From Enhancing Your Membership: Sections, Alexandria, VA, 1993, American Physical Therapy Association.

In addition to the publications listed in Table 4-1, section members share information at an annual **Combined Sections Meeting** in early February. This provides a mechanism for educational and business sessions. Section leadership can then accurately represent the members at other APTA and government arenas.

Assemblies

Assemblies are similar to sections in that they provide a mechanism for members with common interests to meet, confer, and promote their objectives. The differences are that they are composed of members of the same class (category) and may exist at the state and national levels. One exception to the class limitation applies to student and student affiliate members who may combine into one assembly.

This level of organization is relatively new to the APTA. Only two assemblies currently exist: Student Assembly (automatic membership for student and student affiliate classes) and Affiliate Assembly. Each provides an important vehicle for communication and voice for its members.

House of Delegates

The **House of Delegates (HOD)** is the highest policy-making body of the APTA. Officers, directors, and members of the Nominating Committee are elected by the House. Its General Powers, noted in Box 4-4[3], are derived from the Bylaws of the APTA.

Box 4-4

General Powers of the House of Delegates*

The House of Delegates has all legislative and elective powers and authority to determine policies of the Association, including the power to:

A. Amend and repeal these Bylaws;
B. Amend, suspend, or rescind the Standing Rules;
C. Adopt ethical principles and standards to govern the conduct of members of the Association in their roles as physical therapists or physical therapist assistants; and
D. Modify or reverse a decision of the Board of Directors.

*   From Bylaws of the American Physical Therapy Association, Phys Ther 74(10):969-977, 1994.

The HOD is composed of delegates from all chapters, sections, and assemblies. Representation is proportionate; however, the complex formula for determining the size of the House ensures that the total number of delegates will always be slightly above 400. In addition, each chapter has at least two delegates, each section one delegate, and each assembly two delegates. Delegates from sections and assemblies and members of the Board of Directors may speak and make motions, but do not have the right to vote.

In accordance with the Bylaws, the annual business meeting of the APTA is the HOD meeting. This generally occurs in June, spans three days, and is held in conjunction with an **annual conference.** The annual conference continues for another two to three days and includes an extensive program of presentations and activities.

Ad hoc committee and task forces, in addition to standing committees, may be created by the HOD to address issues which it deems important. When this occurs, definite charges and time lines are stipulated in the motion which created the unit.

Board of Directors

Six officers of the APTA and nine directors constitute the **Board of Directors (BOD).** The officers are President, Vice President, Secretary, Treasurer, Speaker of the House of Delegates, and Vice Speaker of the House of Delegates. The duty of the BOD is to carry out the mandates and policies established by the HOD. Full meetings generally occur in November and March.

The Board and House must work closely together for effective operation of the APTA. While the House of Delegates establishes the policies and positions of the APTA, the Board of Directors, elected by the House, communicates these issues to internal and external personnel/agencies. This is an important representative function of the BOD.

Similar to the HOD, the BOD may create ad hoc committees and task forces to carry out its business. These will also have specific charges and time lines. In addition, the BOD may establish councils to respond to unique service needs of the APTA.

Staff

The organizational chart in Figure 4-2 indicates that APTA staff serve the organization at multiple levels. During any business hour, a member (or non-member) can call the APTA headquarters in Alexandria, Virginia, at a toll free number (1-800-999-APTA) and speak to one of over 125 staff members. This direct benefit is important to access information and services. Staff also provide guidance for activities of the chapters, sections, and assemblies, and for the operation of the House of Delegates and Board of Directors.

Key staff members also provide important representative functions to outside agencies similar to duties of the Board of Directors. This is particularly true for the Chief Executive Officer and Senior Vice Presidents. These individuals are responsible for the following Divisions: Executive; Communications; Education; Finance/Administrative; Governance, Components, and Meetings; Health Policy and Practice; and Research, Analysis and Development.

Affiliated Units

In addition to the components identified in Figure 4-2, several related units were created by the House of Delegates or exist independent of the APTA. In both cases, these agencies function to directly benefit the APTA. These units are briefly described below.

Special Interest Groups (SIGs). Special Interest Groups exist at multiple levels of the APTA. Bylaws authorize SIGs within a chapter, section, and assembly. This provides an opportunity for members in one of these components to further organize into smaller specialty areas. For example, the Section on Education has three SIGs for academic administrators, clinical faculty, and academic faculty. Participation in any SIG is voluntary.

American Board of Physical Therapy Specialties (ABPTS). This unit was created by the House of Delegates in 1978 to provide a formal mechanism to recognize physical therapists with advanced knowledge, skills, and experience in a special area of practice. A specialization program was established to achieve board certification and enhance the quality of care in the specialty area. Participation in the program is voluntary; however, no physical therapist shall present her/himself as a "Board Certified Clinical Specialist" unless that individual has successfully completed the certification process.

Each specialty area must be approved by the House of Delegates; however, criteria for each area are established by the ABPTS. Seven specialty areas have been approved (Table 4-2). Two additional ones are under consideration in the areas of Oncology and Obstetrics and Gynecology.

Table 4-2: Approved Specialty Areas in Physical Therapy

Specialty Area	Year Approved
Cardiopulmonary Physical Therapy	1981
Clinical Electrophysiologic Physical Therapy	1982
Geriatric Physical Therapy	1989
Neurologic Physical Therapy	1982
Orthopaedic Physical Therapy	1981
Pediatric Physical Therapy	1981
Sports Physical Therapy	1981

In order to be recognized as a "Board Certified Clinical Specialist," a physical therapist must pass a written exam and present the following qualifications: (1) specified minimum number of hours of clinical practice in past 10 years; (2) competence in administration, consultation, or communication; (3) evidence of review of scientific literature and research process; (4) experience in teaching; and (5) any other criteria specific to the specialty area. The first three specialists were recognized in 1985 in the area of cardiopulmonary physical therapy. Since then, there has been a 25 percent increase in the number of specialists recognized annually so that 1031 existed in 1994.

Commission on Accreditation in Physical Therapy Education (CAPTE). This unit is responsible for evaluating and accrediting professional (entry-level) physical therapy and physical therapist assistant education programs. It is recognized by the US Department of Education and Commission on Recognition of Postsecondary Accreditation. The CAPTE is composed of 17 members including physical therapy educators and practitioners, administrators from institutions of higher education, public representatives, and a physician. (See Chapter 1 for a historical account of accreditation in physical therapy.)

The relationship between the APTA and CAPTE is integrated, yet technically independent. A Department of Accreditation within the APTA manages the accreditation program. However, the CAPTE reviews the data and determines the accreditation status of each educational program. Moreover, the CAPTE establishes the evaluative criteria for the accreditation decisions. It derives its recognition from the House of Delegates which returns the ultimate authority to the APTA.

BENEFITS OF BELONGING

There are intangible and tangible benefits of belonging to the APTA. The intangible benefits relate to the commitment to the profession of physical therapy. As the recognized voice for this profession in the United States, it is appropriate for physical therapists, physical therapist assistants, and students to join the APTA. Through the organizational structure described previously, members are represented in a wide variety of public and governmental areas.

The tangible benefits are identified in Table 4-3[1] and briefly described here. Publications serve as formal communications among members. Research in the profession and newsworthy items are included. Information is made available through on-line computer services, staff contacts, and reference lists. An internet address (HTTP://APTA.EDOC.COM/APTA/) has just been developed to provide widespread access to current information. Professional development occurs through interaction at local, state, and national levels. Specialist certification is available through a recognized board certification process. Insurance and business services provide low cost group programs endorsed by the APTA. Legislative efforts are provided through lobbying, direct contacts and a strong infrastructure to represent the members.

Table 4-3: Benefits of Belonging to the APTA*

Area of Activity	Example
Publications	• Physical Therapy • PT - Magazine of Physical Therapy • PT Bulletin
Information	• APTA-NET (on-line computer service) • Staff consultation on research and practice issues • Bibliographies • Medline searches • Archival resources
Professional Development	• Networking and education through districts, chapters, sections and assemblies
Specialist Certification	• Board certification by ABPTS
Insurance and Business Services	• Professional liability insurance • Visa and MasterCard • Home and auto loans and mortgage program • Student loan program • Short-term major medical coverage • Group term life insurance • Student health plan
Legislative efforts	• Health care reform • Direct access • Reimbursement

*   From APTA Benefits of Belonging, Alexandria, VA, 1994, American Physical Therapy Association.

Special incentives are provided for student membership. Fees for membership and participation in activities are generally 10-25 percent of the cost for an active member. In addition, a three-year dues increment to convert from student to active member after graduation (from 1/3 to 2/3 to full) eases the financial transition to the higher dues level.

RELATED
ORGANIZATIONS

The APTA is a very active organization both internally and externally. It is important to note and describe some key external organizations which have a direct impact on the APTA or the profession of physical therapy. In some cases, APTA serves as a member unit in these agencies.

Foundation for Physical Therapy Research

This body was established in 1979 by an act of the APTA HOD. It was created to promote and provide financial support for research and scholarship in physical therapy. As an independent entity, its governing body is separate from the APTA and consists of clinicians, researchers, and business leaders. Since its inception, it has provided nearly $4 million in awards for research and education. Awards are distributed in the areas of general research (maximum of $30,000 annually for two years), doctoral research (maximum of $15,000 annually for four years), as well as a variety of special scholarships (minority students, students committed to cultural diversity, and physically challenged students). More recently, the Foundation established the first Physical Therapy Clinical Research Center located at the University of Iowa and identified four priority areas to fund national conferences and research: work-related injuries, geriatrics, sports injuries, and catastrophic injury. Through these comprehensive programs, the Foundation promotes clinically focused research to improve the practice and cost effectiveness of physical therapy.

Federation of State Boards of Physical Therapy

This independent agency has been instrumental in coordinating activity among each of the state boards which regulates physical therapy. Two areas of attention have been the licensing exam and violations of ethical conduct. Regarding the exams, the APTA contracts with an outside agency, Professional Examination Services, to administer the national licensing exam. The Federation has been involved in revising the exam and standardizing passing criteria among the states. Concerning ethical conduct, the Federation has surveyed state boards to identify common areas of violations and ensure that proper procedures exist to review cases of alleged violations.

American Academy of Physical Therapists

This organization was founded in 1989 to address the professional needs and concerns of African Americans and other minorities in regards to the profession and practices of physical therapy. Its mission includes encouraging minority students to pursue careers in the allied health professions. The Academy also promotes clinical research which relates to the health of minorities. Business and educational programs have been conducted at its annual conferences.

United Societies of Physiotherapists, Inc.

This is another organization which consists of and represents physical therapists. Membership qualifications are not limited to one group; however, most of the members are engaged in private practice. The purpose is to improve the professional status of the "licensed physiotherapist," create fair reimbursement rates and methods, and maintain the highest level of competency in physical therapy services. It is composed of independent physical therapy associations in several states and at-large members, who send representatives to an Executive Board. The United Societies retains a legislative representative and legal counsel and has been active in legislative efforts regarding the practice of physical therapy.

World Confederation of Physical Therapy

This organization represents physical therapy on a global level. Member organizations are from 64 nations around the world, including the APTA. In addition to annual business meetings, an international congress is held every four years to provide a forum to share information and to collaborate on mutual goals.

Triallance

The Triallance was formed in 1988 and consists of the APTA, the American Occupational Therapy Association, and the American Speech, Language and Hearing Association. This organization meets three times per year to discuss issues of mutual concern. Current issues include professional ethics, the Americans with Disabilities Act, health care reform, and managed care. This unified voice provides greater strength when interacting with governmental and private agencies.

SUMMARY

This chapter described the purposes, infrastructure, benefits, and organizations related to the American Physical Therapy Association. Purposes of the APTA include serving the public and its members to enhance the profession and practice of physical therapy. Its governing bodies are organized into three levels: local (districts), state (chapters), and national (House of Delegates and Board of Directors). Opportunities for participation in areas of special interest exist in sections, assemblies, and special interest groups. Staff members are readily available to support the organization at all levels and interact with external agencies. Benefits of belonging include outcomes which are intangible (professional commitment) and tangible (publications, meetings, computer services, specialist certification, low-cost insurance and business services, and legislative efforts). Other related organizations exist which further promote physical therapy and the APTA participates in these either through direct membership or interaction. Through its purpose, organization, and activities, the APTA provides widespread opportunities and strong representation for the profession and practice of physical therapy.

References

1. APTA benefits of belonging, Alexandria, VA, 1994, American Physical Therapy Association.

2. APTA mission statement, HOD 06-93-05-05, Alexandria, VA, 1993, American Physical Therapy Association.

3. Bylaws of the American Physical Therapy Association, Phys Ther 74(10):969-977, 1994.

4. Enhancing your membership: sections, Alexandria, VA, 1993, American Physical Therapy Association.

5. 1996 goals that represent the priorities of the Association, HOD 06-95-15-27, Alexandria, VA, 1995, American Physical Therapy Association.

6. Policy on APTA mission statement, HOD 06-93-06-07, Alexandria, VA, 1993, American Physical Therapy Association.

7. Standing rules of the American Physical Therapy Association, Phys Ther 74(10):978-980, 1994.

Suggested Readings

Program Directors' APTA Resource Book, Alexandria, VA, 1994, American Physical Therapy Association. This loose-leaf bound resource book was distributed to all physical therapist and physical therapist assistant program directors in 1993. It is updated annually and therefore, contains current information and documents in the areas of background and structure of the APTA, standards and guidelines, benefits, student membership, and post graduation activities.

Review Questions

1. Select at least three components of the APTA Mission Statement and apply them to Fig. 4-2, indicating at what level of APTA each goal should be most logically tackled. There may easily be more than one answer!

2. Apply the goals listed in Box 4-3 to the various levels of APTA's organizational structure (Fig. 4-1), comparing these to your applications in Question 1 and to the definitions of various APTA components, given in this chapter.

3. What is the difference between an assembly and SIG? How do they differ in function and membership?

4. Write to one of the physical therapy organizations besides the APTA to discern differences in scope and function. What advantage do they offer over membership in the APTA alone?

Chapter 5

Laws, Regulations, and Policies

Michael A. Pagliarulo

"No one in the medical business is immune from that harbinger of bad news—the postman delivering word of a liability suit. Not the most judicious physician. Not the most conscientious anesthetist. Not even the most devoted registered physical therapist."

John Scanlon

KEY TERMS

Code of Ethics
common law
law
malpractice
negligence
non-compete clause
policy
practice acts
regulations
Respondeat Superior
Standards of Ethical Conduct for the Physical Therapist Assistant
Standards of Practice for Physical Therapy
statute

Previous chapters presented the evolution, definition, and scope of activities for physical therapists and physical therapist assistants. The focus was on what these individuals *do*.

However, it is just as important, if not more important, to learn about the restrictions to practice as it is to learn about the scope of activities. This chapter describes those restrictions—that is, what a physical therapist or physical therapist assistant *cannot do*. Similarities and differences among laws, regulations, and policies which affect physical therapy will be presented with examples to demonstrate the principles and highlight significant documents. Because of the introductory level of this text, it is beyond the scope of this chapter to present the details regarding medico-legal aspects of practice. The reader is referred to other sources for this level of detail.

GENERAL
DESCRIPTION

What are laws, regulations and policies? Who makes them? What is their purpose and impact on physical therapy? What are the consequences of breaking one of them? These issues and others will be described in this section.

Definition, Purpose, and Impact

Laws, regulations, and policies should not be seen as negative influences on the profession and practice of physical therapy. On the contrary, they exist to serve their constituents and protect the public. Each will be considered here in more detail.

Law. A **law** is "that which is laid down, ordained, or established."[1] Two types of laws affecting physical therapy are statutory and common. A **statute** is "a formal written enactment of a legislative body, whether federal, state, city, or county."[1] It may declare a position or right, mandate a program, or enable an activity. **Common laws** are created by court decision. These do not involve legislative action, but result from legal cases and decisions by juries and judges regarding the outcome of the issue. These differences not withstanding, in the context of this chapter, laws will refer collectively to both statutory and common law.

Laws are generally created in the public's interest. They establish and protect rights, direct activities, and provide opportunities for programs. Regarding physical therapy, they establish qualifications for practice within their jurisdiction ("practice acts"). In this way, they prevent dishonest or unqualified individuals from rendering physical therapy services. They also ensure that health care will be provided to certain populations and that public facilities and services are accessible to all individuals including those with disabilities (e.g., Medicare and Americans with Disabilities Act).

Laws are binding on the individuals who reside or conduct activities within the jurisdiction of the body which created the law. For example, Medicare is a federal law (part of the Social Security Act) and applies to all citizens within the United States. In contrast, physical therapy practice acts are state laws which regulate the practice of physical therapy within that state only.

Significant differences among state laws can and do exist. Practitioners must be aware of and understand the opportunities and limitations which vary from one state to the next. This is particularly important for individuals who may reside close to a state boundary and practice in both states. What is legal in one state may be illegal in the adjacent state.

What are the consequences of breaking a law? They vary from a minor fine or restriction to a serious sentence such as imprisonment or in extreme cases the death penalty in states where capital punishment is permitted. Allegations of illegal activity may be initiated by law enforcement officials or citizens through suits.

Regulation. Regulations are not laws, but are closely associated. They "are issued by various governmental departments to carry out the intent of the law."[1] They are created by administrative units, not enacted by legislatures and serve to interpret and implement laws.

Once again using the examples of Medicare and state practice acts, regulations associated with Medicare are approved by the Health Care Financing Administration (HCFA)[10]; those affecting state practice acts are the responsibility of state boards of physical therapy (or similar units). In many cases, the regulations become more important to the daily practice of physical therapy than the laws because the former will specifically identify what must or can be done. For example, although Medicare entitles health care to older adults, physical therapy services are limited by number of visits and dollar amounts. These cost saving measures do not always provide maximum benefit to the patient.

It is clear that members of the physical therapy profession must be current in understanding laws and regulations. Furthermore, it is in their best interest and that of the public to understand and participate in the appropriate processes for changing laws and regulations.

The consequences of regulatory infractions can be serious, although not as severe as those incurred by breaking a law. Generally, an administrative agency investigates the alleged regulatory infraction and imposes a punishment if the infraction is found to be true. This may range from a written reprimand, to a fine and loss of license to practice in that jurisdiction.

Policy. A **policy** is a plan or course of action which is designed to influence and determine decisions. As defined by and applied to the American Physical Therapy Association (APTA), it is "a decision which obligates actions or subsequent decisions on similar matters."[4] Policies are separate from procedures which identify and describe the actions required to implement the policies.

Policies are established by a variety of organizations including governmental agencies, professional organizations, and businesses. They set standards by which the members of that organization must abide.

While it is universally understood physical therapy practice and services must be rendered legally, the policies which affect those services are not as widely known. Three important origins for these policies are the APTA, insurance carriers, and employers. Membership in the APTA is voluntary; however, all members must abide by its policies such as the Code of Ethics for physical therapists or Standards of Ethical Conduct for the Physical Therapist Assistant. Adherence to policies of insurance carriers is essential for reimbursement for services provided to each covered patient. Finally, employees must abide by policies approved by the employer assuming, of course, that they are fair and equitable.

If one breaches a policy, the consequences vary according to the controlling agency and situation. Administrators may independently review the case and render a judgment or a procedure may be available for an administrative hearing. Judgments may range from no consequences to expulsion from the organization (including firing), or refusal to reimburse for services rendered.

EXAMPLES
AFFECTING
PHYSICAL
THERAPY

Examples of laws, regulations, and policies which have a direct impact on the practice of physical therapy are described here. This section is neither a comprehensive review nor a detailed description of the mandates which affect physical therapy, but provides a sample for demonstration purposes. Malpractice is also briefly described to highlight its important legal impact on practice.

Laws

Practice Acts. Perhaps the laws which are most critical to physical therapy are the **practice acts** enacted by each state. These laws regulate practice by stating the conditions to be met to obtain a license to practice within that jurisdiction. They generally define the practice, list the qualifications needed to practice, and may address certain responsibilities such as supervision of personnel or requirements to maintain a current license.

Practice acts are instrumental in identifying what a physical therapist (PT) or physical therapist assistant (PTA) can or cannot do. As noted elsewhere in this text, PTs are licensed in all states, whereas PTAs are regulated (license, certification, or otherwise) in only 41 states (see Chapter 3). This has important implications regarding the scope of activities permitted for each level of health care provider and the supervisory relationship described by law.

Another specific responsibility addressed in the practice acts is whether or not the PT may practice using direct access. This is currently legal in 30 states; however, certain conditions may apply, such as: (1) minimum number of years of practice, (2) referral to a physician within a certain period of time or number of visits, and (3) distinction between direct access evaluation and treatment. This issue is further compounded by regulations and policies from other agencies which require a physician's signature for reimbursement (e.g., Medicare and insurance carriers).

The most important factor to recognize regarding this type of law is the real and potential variability among the states. For this reason, the APTA has approved a model definition to be used in practice acts to provide a standard to describe the profession and practice of physical therapy (see Chapter 1).

Federal legislation. Three examples of federal legislation (laws) that affect physical therapy services are: (1) the Social Security Act (Medicare), (2) PL 94-142 (Education of All Handicapped Children Act), and (3) Americans with Disabilities Act (ADA). The first two have direct impact, and the second has indirect impact.

Medicare and PL 94-142 mandate services for certain age populations, namely the elderly and children. Medicare provides payment for certain health care costs including physical therapy, while PL 94-142 provides special services including physical therapy to children. The result has been an increase in physical therapy services provided to both age groups and a shift in the setting where the services are provided. For example, physical therapy services have expanded in nursing homes and extended care facilities. They have also become part of the school environment for children as provided by PL 94-142 (as amended by PL 99-457). (See also Chapter 7 for more on PL 94-142 and 99-457).

In response to the ADA, which was created to eliminate discrimination against individuals with disabilities, physical therapists have been involved as consultants to rectify architectural barriers in the community and work place. Access to buildings and service areas (e.g., dining areas, restrooms) must be available to individuals with disabilities. Modifications may include ramps, wider doorways, automatic doors, and elevators, as well as lower counter areas, and mirrors. Physical therapists are familiar with the functional needs of these individuals and provide advice regarding environmental modifications.

Malpractice. This area of law is more closely related to common law (court decisions) than statutory law (legislation). However, it is included here because it has direct impact on physical therapy practice. Professional liability insurance, while not required for practice, is prudent to protect against losses from malpractice suits which might arise for reasons noted below.

Malpractice refers to injuries or wrongful behavior which an individual (patient/client) sustains from a provider (PT or PTA). **Negligence** is the specific term used to describe the act. This involves: (1) a duty, (2) breach of duty, and (3) damage to the individual's (patient/client) person or property.[6] Claims brought against physical therapists usually involve inadequate monitoring of the patient resulting in burns, infections, opening of wounds, soft tissue tears, and falls.[10] Other reasons include faulty equipment, failure to refer or follow physician's orders, and sexual misconduct.

Supervisory and employer-employee relationships become significant in malpractice suits. A concept known as the doctrine of **Respondeat Superior** places the service responsibility on the supervisor or employer. Literally translated as "let the superior respond", this doctrine is based upon the principle that the master (employer/supervisor) is responsible for the acts/liabilities of the servant (employee/supervisee) while providing services under the work relationship.[6] This implies that PTs may be named in a malpractice suit as an employer (private practice) or supervisor. While professional liability insurance is wise, it is more effective to take preventive action in one's practice to avoid malpractice litigation.

Regulations

Regulations frequently have a greater impact than the law itself. They guide, direct, and limit actions which implement the laws. Two examples affecting physical therapy practice are state regulations on professional conduct and HCFA regulations concerning Medicare.

A license to practice physical therapy in a state provides opportunities but also brings responsibilities. The PT must abide by regulations which may apply to all professions licensed in that state. These generally protect the public from inappropriate acts such as fraud, abuse, sexual misconduct, misrepresentation, or delegating to unqualified personnel. As noted above, an infraction in one of these areas may result in a suspended or revoked license.

The HCFA regulations are extensive and beyond the scope of this chapter. Conceptually, however, they provide limits to the physical therapy services available through Medicare and require extensive documentation of services for reimbursement. While the intent to control health care costs is appropriate, the limits are occasionally unrealistic. For this reason, the APTA has been attempting to amend the regulations in the best interests of the consumer.

Policies

Policies are different from laws and regulations in that they generally do not have legal implications. They do, however, directly influence practice as described in the areas of the APTA, insurance carriers, and employers.

APTA. The APTA is the professional organization recognized to represent the profession of physical therapy in the United States. It establishes policies for its members through the House of Delegates and Board of Directors (see Chapter 4). These are reviewed and updated annually. While many of these are internal in nature, those that identify standards of ethics and practice affect the public and are described below.

Two policies of the APTA which establish standards for ethical behavior are the **Code of Ethics**[2] (Box 5-1) and **Standards of Ethical Conduct for the Physical Therapist Assistant**[8] (Box 5-2). These documents pertain to the PT and PTA, respectively. Companion documents, Guide for Professional Conduct (for Code) and Guide for Conduct of the Affiliate Member (for Standards) provide interpretations for each item in the specific policy.

Box 5-1

Code of Ethics*

Preamble
This Code of Ethics sets forth ethical principles for the physical therapy profession. Members of this profession are responsible for maintaining and promoting ethical practice. This Code of Ethics, adopted by the American Physical Therapy Association, shall be binding on physical therapists who are members of the Association.

Principle 1
Physical therapists respect the rights and dignity of all individuals.

Principle 2
Physical therapists comply with the laws and regulations governing the practice of physical therapy.

Principle 3
Physical therapists accept responsibility for the exercise of sound judgment.

Principle 4
Physical therapists maintain and promote high standards for physical therapy practice, education, and research.

Principle 5
Physical therapists seek remuneration for their services that is deserved and reasonable.

Principle 6
Physical therapists provide accurate information to the consumer about the profession and about those services they provide.

Principle 7
Physical therapists accept the responsibility to protect the public and the profession from unethical, incompetent, or illegal acts.

Principle 8
Physical therapists participate in efforts to address the health needs of the public.

Adopted by the House of Delegates
June 1981
Amended June 1987
Amended June 1991

*   From Code of Ethics, HOD 06-91-05-05, Alexandria, VA, 1991, American Physical Therapy Association. Reprinted with permission from the American Physical Therapy Association.

Box 5-2

Standards of Ethical Conduct for the Physical Therapist Assistant*

Preamble
Physical therapist assistants are responsible for maintaining and promoting high standards of conduct. These Standards of Ethical Conduct for the Physical Therapist Assistant shall be binding on physical therapist assistants who are affiliate members of the Association.

Standard 1
Physical therapist assistants provide services under the supervision of a physical therapist.

Standard 2
Physical therapist assistants respect the rights and dignity of all individuals.

Standard 3
Physical therapist assistants maintain and promote high standards in the provision of services, giving the welfare of the patients their highest regard.

Standard 4
Physical therapist assistants provide services within the limits of the law.

Standard 5
Physical therapist assistants make those judgments that are commensurate with their qualifications as physical therapist assistants.

Standard 6
Physical therapist assistants accept the responsibility to protect the public and the profession from unethical, incompetent, or illegal acts.

Adopted by House of Delegates
June 1982
Amended June 1991

* From Standards of Ethical Conduct for the Physical Therapist Assistant, HOD 06-91-06-07, Alexandria, VA, 1991, American Physical Therapy Association. Reprinted with permission from the American Physical Therapy Association.

The Judicial Committee of the APTA is responsible for conducting hearings regarding alleged violations of ethical conduct. It follows with precision the steps it has outlined in The Procedural Document on Disciplinary Action of the American Physical Therapy Association which directs activity at the chapter level before the case proceeds to the Committee. The most common reasons for Committee hearings are to review allegations of inappropriate delegation, unprofessional conduct (e.g., misleading ads), and sexual misconduct.[3] Decisions of the Committee have ranged from dismissal of the case to expulsion from the APTA.

Another significant document which guides the provision of physical therapy services is the **Standards of Practice for Physical Therapy**[9] (Fig. 5-1). This document addresses the administration of services and plan of care, as well as the education, research, community, and ethical/legal responsibilities of the PT. It emulates the high standards of the profession as established by the APTA.

Insurance Carriers. It is impractical if not impossible to reconstruct the policies established by all insurance carriers which provide reimbursement for physical therapy services. The important issue is to identify, understand, and adhere to the pertinent policies to provide the necessary care and receive appropriate payment for services. In many cases, mechanisms for appeals for unusual circumstances (e.g., medical complications) are provided; however, this is considered an exception, not the rule.

Extensive variety in forms and policies has resulted in time-consuming responsibilities in documentation. Computer technology has provided a great deal of efficiency to this process, but effectiveness remains dependent upon following the policies and procedures appropriately.

Employers. A final area worth addressing regarding policies pertains to those established by employers. Two examples are the job description and conditions of employment.

When securing a new job or position, each employee should request and review the job description for the position. This will include not only the title and primary responsibilities, but also specific qualifications and the individual to whom the person in such a position reports. These are important to recognize before accepting a position.

Conditions of employment will vary according to the setting. However, two issues are relevant to new and experienced PTs/PTAs. The shortage of PTs and PTAs has resulted in aggressive marketing campaigns by potential employers. These have included attractive scholarships for students to help defray the cost of education. In return, the sponsoring institution requires a service commitment immediately after graduation. Many of these arrangements are mutually beneficial to the parties involved; however, students should pause before committing to lofty opportunities. The APTA has become concerned and established a policy which provides guidelines to students for consideration before signing a service-related scholarship[5] (Box 5-3). Students should fully understand the nature of the position, practice environment, employment conditions, and perhaps seek legal counsel before agreeing to the offer.

American Physical Therapy Association

STANDARDS OF PRACTICE FOR PHYSICAL THERAPY

PREAMBLE

The physical therapy profession is committed to provide an optimum level of care and to strive for excellence in practice. The House of Delegates of the American Physical Therapy Association, as the responsible body representing this profession, attests to this commitment by adopting, publishing, disseminating, and promoting the application of the following *Standards of Practice for Physical Therapy*. These *Standards of Practice* are the profession's statement of conditions and performances which are essential for quality physical therapy. They provide a foundation for assessment of physical therapy practice.

ADMINISTRATION OF THE PHYSICAL THERAPY SERVICE

I. Purposes and Goals

A written statement of purposes and goals exists for the physical therapy service which reflects the needs of the individuals served, the physical therapy personnel, the facility, and the community.

- ◆ Define scope and limitation of service.
- ◆ Contain current description of purpose.
- ◆ List objectives and goals of services provided.
- ◆ Are appropriate for the population (community) served.
- ◆ Provide a mechanism for annual review.

II. Organizational Plan

A written organizational plan exists for the physical therapy service.

- ◆ Describes the interrelationships within the overall organization.
- ◆ Provides for direction of service by a physical therapist.
- ◆ Defines supervisory functions within the program/service.
- ◆ Reflects current personnel functions.

III. Policies and Procedures

Written policies and procedures, which reflect the operation of the service, exist and are consistent with the purposes and goals of the physical therapy service.

- ◆ Address pertinent information about the following:
  - ◆ Clinical education
  - ◆ Clinical research
  - ◆ Criteria for access to, initiation, and termination of care
  - ◆ Equipment maintenance
  - ◆ Fire and disaster
  - ◆ Infection control
  - ◆ Job descriptions
  - ◆ Medical emergencies
  - ◆ Patient care policies and protocols
  - ◆ Patient rights
  - ◆ Personnel-related policies
  - ◆ Position descriptions
  - ◆ Quality assurance
  - ◆ Record keeping
  - ◆ Safety
  - ◆ Staff orientation
  - ◆ Supervisory relationships
- ◆ Meet the requirements of external agencies and state law.
- ◆ Meet the requirements of the overall organization.
- ◆ Be reviewed on a regular basis.

IV. Administration

A physical therapist shall be responsible for the direction of the physical therapy service.

- ◆ Assures that the service is consistent with established purposes and goals.
- ◆ Assures that the service is provided in accordance with established policies and procedures.
- ◆ Assures compliance with local, state, and federal requirements.
- ◆ Complies with current APTA *Standards of Practice* and *Guide for Professional Conduct*.
- ◆ Reviews and updates policies and procedures as appropriate.
- ◆ Provides appropriate education, training, and review of physical therapy support personnel.

V. Staffing

The physical therapy personnel are qualified and sufficient in number to achieve the purposes and goals of the physical therapy service.

- ◆ Meets legal requirements regarding licensure and/or certification of appropriate personnel.
- ◆ Provides expertise appropriate to the case mix.
- ◆ Provides adequate staff to patient ratio.
- ◆ Provides adequate support staff to professional staff.

VI. Physical Setting

1. The physical setting is designed to provide a safe and effective environment that facilitates the achievement of the purposes and goals of the physical therapy service.

- ◆ Meets all applicable legal requirements for health and safety.
- ◆ Meets space needs appropriate for the number and type of patients served.

2. Equipment is safe and sufficient to achieve the purposes and goals of the physical therapy service.

- ◆ Meets all applicable legal requirements for health and safety.
- ◆ Meets equipment needs appropriate for the number and type of patients served.
- ◆ Provides for routine safety inspection of equipment by a qualified individual.

VII. Fiscal Affairs

Fiscal planning and management of the physical therapy service are based upon sound accounting principles.

- ◆ Include preparation and use of a budget.
- ◆ Conform to legal requirements.
- ◆ Are accurately recorded and reported.
- ◆ Provide for optimum use of resources.
- ◆ Include a plan for audit control.
- ◆ Establish the basis for a fee schedule consistent with cost of service and within customary norms of fair and reasonable.

VIII. Quality Assurance

A written plan exists for the assessment of, and action to assure, the quality and appropriateness of the physical therapy service.

- ◆ Provides for a current written plan for assessment of the service.
- ◆ Provides evidence of ongoing review, evaluation of the service.
- ◆ Resolves identified problems.
- ◆ Is consistent with requirements of external agencies.

continued

Fig. 5-1. Standards of Practice for Physical Therapy. A policy of the House of Delegates, APTA, which provides standards to emulate in the delivery of physical therapy services. (From Standards of Practice for Physical Therapy, HOD 06-91-21-25, Alexandria, VA, 1991, American Physical Therapy Association. Reprinted with permission from the American Physical Therapy Association.)

IX. Staff Development

A written plan exists which provides for appropriate ongoing development of staff.

◆ Is reflected by evidence of ongoing education or attendance at continuing education activities.

PROVISION OF CARE

X. Informed Consent

The physical therapist obtains the patient's informed consent in accordance with jurisdictional law before initiating physical therapy.

XI. Initial Evaluation

The physical therapist performs and records an initial evaluation and interprets results to determine appropriate care for the individual.

◆ Is initiated prior to treatment.

◆ Is performed by the physical therapist in a timely manner.

◆ Is documented, dated, and signed by the physical therapist who performed the evaluation.

◆ Identifies physical therapy needs of the client.

◆ Includes pertinent information of the following:
  ◆ History
  ◆ Diagnosis
  ◆ Problem
  ◆ Complications and precautions
  ◆ Physical status
  ◆ Functional status
  ◆ Critical behavior/mentation
  ◆ Social/environmental needs

◆ Provides sufficient data to establish time-related goals.

◆ The physical therapist shall render care within the scope of the physical therapist's education and experience. Appropriate referral to other practitioners shall be made when necessary.

◆ The physical therapist utilizes objective measures to establish a baseline at the time of the initial evaluation.

◆ Is documented, dated, and signed by the physical therapist who performed the evaluation.

XII. Plan of Care

1. The physical therapist establishes and records a plan of care for the individual based on the results of the evaluation.

◆ Includes realistic goals and expected outcome.

◆ Is based on identified needs.

◆ Includes effective treatment, frequency, and duration.

◆ Recommends appropriate coordination of care with other professionals/services.

◆ Is documented, dated, and signed by the physical therapist who established the plan of care.

2. The physical therapist involves the individual/significant other in the planning, implementation, and revision of the treatment program.

3. The physical therapist plans for discharge of the individual, taking into consideration goal achievement, and provides for appropriate follow-up or referral.

XIII. Treatment

1. The physical therapist provides or delegates and supervises the physical therapy treatment consistent with the results of the evaluation and plan of care.

◆ Is under the ongoing personal care or supervision of the physical therapist.

◆ Reflects that delegated responsibilities are commensurate with the qualifications of the physical therapy personnel.

◆ Is altered in accordance with changes in individual status.

◆ Is provided at a level consistent with current physical therapy practice.

2. The physical therapist records, on an ongoing basis, treatment rendered, progress, and change in status relative to the plan of care.

XIV. Reevaluation

The physical therapist reevaluates the individual and modifies the plan of care as indicated.

◆ Is performed by the physical therapist in a timely manner.

◆ Reflects that the individual's progress is reassessed relative to initial evaluation and plan of care.

◆ Is documented, dated, and signed by the physical therapist who performed the evaluation.

EDUCATION

XV. Professional Development

The physical therapist is responsible for his/her individual professional development and continued competence in physical therapy.

XVI. Student

The physical therapist participates in the education of physical therapy students and other student health professionals.

RESEARCH

XVII. The physical therapist utilizes research findings in practice and encourages or participates in research activities.

COMMUNITY RESPONSIBILITY

XVIII. The physical therapist participates in community activities to promote community health.

LEGAL/ETHICAL

XIX. Legal

The physical therapist fulfills all the legal requirements of the jurisdictions regulating the practice of physical therapy.

XX. Ethical

The physical therapist practices according to the *Code of Ethics* of the American Physical Therapy Association.

American Physical Therapy Association
1111 North Fairfax Street, Alexandria, VA 22314-1488

A-3/1000/6-92

Box 5-3

Guidelines for Student and Employer Contracts*

Guidelines for fairness in offering student financial assistance in exchange for a promise of future employment:

1. Notification by the employer if the place of employment may be in an isolated area or as a solo practitioner such that the new graduate will not have ready access to mentoring and regular collegial relationships or any resources for professional growth and development.
2. Disclosure by the employer of ownership of the practice.
3. Notification by the employer to the student if the practice is involved in any situation in which a referring practitioner can profit as a result of referring patients for physical therapy and notification that the American Physical Therapy Association is opposed to such situations.
4. Student awareness of any potential future tax obligations that may be incurred upon graduation as the result of deferred income.
5. The agreement must not, in any way, interfere with the process and planning of the student's professional education.
6. It should be understood that the school is not a party to the agreement and is not bound to any conditions of the agreement.
7. There should be a clearly delineated, fair, and reasonable buy-out provision in which the student understands the legal commitment to pay back the stipend with reasonable interest in the event that there is dissatisfaction or reason for release from the contract on the student's part at any time during the term of the agreement.
8. A no-penalty bailout provision should be provided in the event of change of ownership, but the student may be required to adhere to a reasonable payback schedule.
9. Avoidance of non-compete clauses is recommended, but if there is one, a reasonable limitation of time and distance should be incorporated.
10. A student's interest may best be served by obtaining appropriate counsel prior to signing the contract.

* From Guidelines for Student and Employer Contracts, HOD 06-92-14-28, Alexandria, VA, 1992, American Physical Therapy Association. Reprinted with permission from the American Physical Therapy Association.

Another employment issue which pertains to experienced as well as new practitioners is a **"non-compete clause."** This is a contract between the employer and employee which stipulates certain conditions of practice following *termination* of employment (voluntary or otherwise). The conditions usually identify a minimum length of time and distance within which the former employee *cannot* establish a practice which will compete with the original employer. These are common in the medical profession and have increased in the physical therapy profession as private practices have increased dramatically. At the time of hiring, the policy (contract) may seem unimportant. However, when contested in court, they have been upheld as legally binding agreements.[7]

SUMMARY

The profession and practice of physical therapy is exciting, demanding, and rewarding. Opportunities continue to develop, which makes it all the more crucial that PTs and PTAs adhere to laws, regulations, and policies which govern the delivery of services. Laws are enactments of legislatures; regulations are established by administrative units to interpret these laws; and policies are adopted by organizations. Examples cited in this chapter which influence the profession and practice of physical therapy were taken from federal and state laws/regulations and policies of the APTA and potential employers. Recognition, understanding, and adherence to these enactments is necessary for legal, ethical, and effective practice.

References

1. Black's law dictionary, ed 5, St. Paul, MN, 1990, West Publishing Co.

2. Code of ethics, HOD 06-91-05-05, Alexandria, VA, 1991, American Physical Therapy Association.

3. Complaints of ethical misconduct quadruple during the last ten years, PT Bulletin 9(18):32-33, May 11, 1994.

4. Definitions, BOD 03-92-12-34, Alexandria, VA, 1992, American Physical Therapy Association.

5. Guidelines for student and employer contracts, HOD 06-92-14-28, Alexandria, VA, 1992, American Physical Therapy Association.

6. Hickok RJ: Physical therapy administration and management, ed 2, Baltimore, 1982, Williams and Wilkins.

7. *Sprague and McCune v Davenport,* unpublished decision of the Supreme Court of the State of New York, Rose J, Tompkins County, Index No. 89-510, September 27, 1990.

8. Standards of ethical conduct for the physical therapist assistant, HOD 06-91-06-07, Alexandria, VA, 1991, American Physical Therapy Association.

9. Standards of practice for physical therapy, HOD 06-91-21-25, Alexandria, VA, 1991, American Physical Therapy Association.

10. Walter J: Physical therapy management: an integrated management, St. Louis, 1993, Mosby-Year Book, Inc.

Suggested Readings

Cowdrey ML, Drew M: Basic law for the allied health professions, ed 2, Boston; 1995, Jones and Bartlett Publishers. The text is written for individuals who have minimal knowledge of legal issues as they pertain to the health care setting. Begins with a description of the law and then applies it to practice settings. Includes case studies and a glossary.

House of Delegates policies, Alexandria, VA, 1995, American Physical Therapy Association. Policies adopted by the House of Delegates of the American Physical Therapy Association. Updated annually. Govern the activities of the organization and its members.

Minor MA, Minor SD: Patient care skills, ed 3, Norwalk, CT, 1995, Appleton and Lange. This manual on techniques of patient handling includes a chapter describing the space requirements to comply with the accessibility directives in the Americans with Disabilities Act.

Risk management: an APTA malpractice resource guide, Alexandria, VA, 1995, American Physical Therapy Association. Provides guidelines for physical therapists to prevent malpractice. Includes a series of articles, case scenarios, APTA reprints and policies, and a bibliography.

Review Questions

1. Suggest examples of decisions that would be considered: (a) a *statute,* (b) a *common law decision,* (c) a *regulation,* and (d) a *policy.*

2. Explain the different purposes and effects of a practice act versus federal legislation. Cite examples.

3. Describe how state regulations for professional conduct differ from HCFA regulations.

4. Cite major differences between the "Code of Ethics" and the "Standards of Practice for Physical Therapy."

5. You have been offered a service based scholarship from an Arizona Indian Reservation and from a Chicago inner-city community center. What factors does the APTA suggest considering for choosing whether to accept such scholarships? What should you know before you decide?

Chapter 6

Current Issues

Susan E. Bennett

"The time is now for us to face the current crisis so that we ensure that the horizon ahead of us is not a receding one. The current health crisis should result in the opening of even greater doors for our profession."
Marilyn Moffat, PT, FAPTA

1994 APTA Presidential Address

KEY TERMS

alliance
ambulatory center
continuous quality improvement or total quality management (CQI/TQM)
critical pathways
cross-training
doctorate in physical therapy (DPT)
encroachment
"gatekeeper"
health maintenance organization (HMO)
managed care network
managed care setting
patient-focused care (PFC)
physician-owned physical therapy service (POPTS)
"post-professional" education
preferred providers

"professional" physical therapy education
reimbursement

The issues that currently affect the profession of physical therapy are very similar to those affecting other health care professions. Practice settings, referrals, reimbursement, encroachment, and peer review are being discussed by occupational therapists, physical therapists, respiratory therapists, nurses, and speech therapists. All health care providers are concerned about changes in the delivery of health care that may impinge on their current practice environment.

This chapter will examine how the issues of educational preparation, practice settings, direct access, physician-owned physical therapy services, encroachment, human resources, reimbursement, continuous quality improvement, and research are affecting the profession of physical therapy. The historical perspective will be presented as appropriate, to demonstrate the longevity of some of these issues.

EDUCATIONAL
PREPARATION

Historical Overview

The extent of the educational preparation and degree required to practice physical therapy has been a topic of debate for some time. The physical therapist evolved from the Reconstruction Aides established during World War I (see Chapter 1). These Reconstruction Aides were trained in emergency courses which were phased out at the end of the war. "Standards for Schools of Physical Therapy" published in 1928, was the first recommended course of study for physical therapy. The American Physical Therapy Association (APTA), at that time called the American Physiotherapy Association, was closely involved in the development of these programs until 1936, when the American Medical Association (AMA) assumed responsibility for overseeing the educational preparation.[10] This was initially perceived to be a positive step for the profession, but as it turned out, the AMA limited the input from physical therapists and never revised or updated the curricula until 1955.

The first discussion of academic degree requirements occurred in 1955, when it was determined that if physical therapy education was integrated with a bachelor's degree program, the graduates could receive a bachelor's degree in physical therapy. This was formalized in 1960 by the APTA's House of Delegates. This action provided strong support to move the first professional degree in physical therapy from the certificate to the bachelor's degree. In 1977, the APTA was recognized as an independent accrediting agency, and in 1983 the APTA became the only recognized accrediting agency for physical therapist and physical therapist assistant education programs. The conflict created by the AMA limiting the growth and independence of educational programs for physical therapy was eliminated with the 1977 action.[10]

Professional Level Education

More controversy was to follow; however, when the APTA House of Delegates adopted a policy in 1979 with amendments in 1980 which ruled that "physical therapist professional education be that which results in the awarding of a postbaccalaureate degree";

and "that all physical therapist professional education programs and all developing phys-ical therapist professional educational programs shall comply with this policy by December 31, 1990."[3] Postbaccalaureate education moved the academic preparation of the physical therapist beyond the bachelor's degree and into the master's degree level. By in January, 1994, 55 percent of the physical therapist education programs were at or had received approval to move to the postbaccalaureate level. While this reflects a substantial transition to postbaccalaureate level education, this also indicates that the policy adopted by the House of Delegates in 1979 could not supersede each state's requirements for education and licensure for physical therapists. Each State Education Department is responsible for establishing and regulating the education and practice of licensed profes-sionals. A national organization, such as the APTA, cannot supersede any rules and regu-lations set by each individual State Education Department. The awarding of the bachelor's or master's degree remains a controversy in many regions of the country.

New terminology was adopted by the House of Delegates in June 1993, to differentiate the entry-level education for physical therapists from an advanced preparation in phys-ical therapy. **"Professional" physical therapy education** refers to all academic programs that prepare students for *entry* into the field of physical therapy regardless of the degree. **"Post-Professional" education** is *advanced* education (either at the master's or doctorate level) of a licensed physical therapist.

Education Today

In 1993, a policy was to be presented to the House of Delegates to investigate the **Doctorate in Physical Therapy (DPT)** as the professional degree. Students in this program, though receiving a doctorate degree, would be entry-level graduates in the field of physical therapy. Other doctoral programs have been proposed, but at the post-professional level (an advanced degree for licensed physical therapists). This policy did not reach the House floor for discussion; however, it did generate much discussion outside of the House of Delegates. As previously noted, the policy adopted in 1979 by the House of Delegates could not mandate a postbaccalaureate degree for physical therapy education, so it is believed that the DPT will meet the same fate. Even discussing a DPT as the professional degree seemed premature to many members of the House of Delegates, especially in view of the status of the postbaccalaureate degree.

There are several other questions that are raised regarding the DPT as the professional degree. Will this degree limit the number of graduates in a society already faced with an inadequate number of physical therapists? What additional knowledge would the DPT graduate have beyond the bachelor's prepared or postbaccalaureate prepared graduate? What will the clinical education requirements consist of in a DPT program (one-year internship)? These questions may remain unanswered for some time.

Physical Therapist Assistant

The evolution of the educational requirement for the physical therapist assistant (PTA) was less controversial. Chapter 3 provides a thorough description of the educational preparation of the PTA. The controversy that exists today with PTA education surrounds the attendance and participation of PTAs at continuing education courses offered for physical therapists. The House of Delegates created the PTA and originally defined their role as a technician, though they have evolved and today are referred to as para-professionals. Many physical therapists (PTs) believe that PTAs should be excluded from attending continuing education courses offered for PTs because the PTA academic preparation prepares them to serve in a supportive role. The PTA does not receive academic preparation equivalent to the PT in the theoretical basis for treatment or in the sciences such as gross anatomy (detailed human anatomy), physics, or neuroscience. Without this academic preparation, PTAs may be unable to thoroughly understand concepts provided in continuing education courses for PTs. With a mixed audience, the course instructor might add information to provide the PTAs with the necessary knowledge at the expense of the PTs in the audience.

The problem has become worse by the limited number of continuing education courses specifically offered for the PTA. Many PTAs have developed the background knowledge needed to attend the continuing education courses offered for PTs through their work experience and interaction with physical therapists. The majority of continuing education courses provided continue to offer open enrollment, which means this debate remains unsolved.

PRACTICE SETTINGS

Background

The practice setting for physical therapy is changing based on health care reform and the distribution of reimbursement dollars. Historically, physical therapy evolved to meet the rehabilitative needs of soldiers from the war and children with polio. Most of these individuals needing physical therapy were treated in hospitals or long-term care facilities. As the profession has expanded, physical therapists can be found treating individuals across the life span who display any variety of problems that impair their ability to move and function. Physical therapists evaluate and treat patients/clients in a variety of practice settings: schools, pediatric clinics, rehabilitation centers, outpatient clinics, wellness clinics, nursing homes, Health Maintenance Organizations (HMOs), fitness centers, private practices, and the patient's home.

Ambulatory Centers

Health care reform has also caused a shift in the delivery of care to ambulatory settings. An **ambulatory center** is any facility in which health care is provided on an outpatient basis. The patient is able to walk into the facility, receive health care, and walk out of the facility the same day. Outpatient clinics and HMOs are examples of ambulatory centers. Health care in this environment is less costly to the consumer and the insurance companies overall. Therefore, this type of setting is becoming more common. In fact, respondents to a survey of 6000 active members conducted by the APTA in 1993 reported that 27.4 percent were practicing in a private practice setting, and 25.4 percent reported that they were practicing in a hospital setting (Fig. 2-15B).[1] This was the first time that the majority of physical therapists were not practicing in a hospital setting.

Health Maintenance Organizations

The private practice environment in physical therapy has traditionally consisted of one or more physical therapists who own a practice, and provide physical therapy services.

In many of these private practices, other physical therapists are employed to provide care for the patients. The physical therapy private practice is an ambulatory setting; however, it is limited in that the only service provided is physical therapy. Many of the health care reform proposals are designed to use ambulatory settings that are multi-purpose. A good example of this is the **Health Maintenance Organization (HMO)** which provides all health care services needed under one roof. In an HMO, you can access your physician, nurse practitioner/physician's assistant, and physical therapist as well as the services of the pharmacy, radiology, and laboratories, in one setting.

Health care reform has emphasized the use of HMOs because of the greater accountability for quality care, peer review and cost containment. There are 40 million members in 550 HMOs across the country.[7] This means that a large percent of the population uses health care providers who work in the HMO. For physicians, this has not been a major problem, because many HMOs contract with several physicians, especially in specialty areas. Physicians can contract with the HMO and practice in a managed care environment with the HMO while also maintaining their private practice. Physical therapists, however, are not as highly sought after by the HMO as physicians; so to save cost, the HMO employs (rather than contracts with) physical therapists to provide care to their members. The majority of physical therapists working in this environment do not maintain a separate private practice, so their sole employment is with the HMO.

Managed Care

The HMO is a perfect example of managed care. A **managed care setting** means that the insurance company contracts with health care providers to provide health care to the consumers who subscribe to the insurance plan. Private practitioners in physical therapy may become what is known as **preferred providers** for insurance company X. This means that when a consumer insured by company X needs physical therapy, the insurance company will refer the consumer to its physical therapy preferred provider. The preferred provider is usually selected on the basis of quality of care and cost containment.

Of recent concern is the selection of health care providers in managed care settings. If a physical therapist is a preferred provider in a managed care setting, she/he may be dropped as a provider if the cost for services becomes too high, even if the quality of care remains excellent. This becomes a concern for consumers who want to have access to the best physical therapist for their rehabilitation but are unable to do so due to the insurance company's refusal to pay the physical therapist's rates. Nearly half the HMOs are owned by the eight top insurance companies, so the selection problem can be found in the HMO as well.

Of greater concern is the inability of all physical therapy private practices to become members of a **managed care network.** A managed care network is a group of health care providers that form a professional cooperative relationship for the purpose of referring individuals to health care providers within the network. The intent of the network is to maintain quality standards of practice of all health care providers in the network. Physical therapists in private practice may be denied the opportunity to become a participating provider in managed care networks, even though they meet the same quality standards established for the network. If health care reform continues to move toward managed care, and if the private practitioner is not allowed to join managed care networks, many private practitioners will be forced to close their offices because they will not be eligible for insurance reimbursement.

Alliances

In addition to managed care, the other major change in health care reform is the formation of alliances. An **alliance** is the collaboration of several health care facilities and practices. For example, two hospitals could merge together and form an alliance. By allying together, they can share resources, programs, health care providers, etc. This makes the two hospitals stronger because of the multitude of services that they can provide under the alliance. An alliance could also be formed between a PT private practitioner and a hospital, or between a private practitioner and other health care providers. The purpose of forming an alliance is to ensure the stability and quality of services that are provided, and to market these services to the insurance companies.

Future of Physical Therapists in the Hospital Setting

The American Hospital Association conducted a study in 1992 of 6700 hospitals in the United States regarding vacancy rates of professional staff.[2] More than half of the hospitals responded to the survey. The hospitals reported a decrease in the vacancy rates for 20 of the 26 professions studied. One of those professions that was reported to have a decrease in vacancy was physical therapy. However, the decrease was insignificant at 0.3 percent from 1991 to 1992. According to the report, a 16.3 percent vacancy rate was still reported in physical therapy, with a recruitment period for physical therapists usually exceeding 90 days.

Many hospitals are exploring contracting physical therapy care versus hiring physical therapists as employees of the hospital. The contracts for physical therapy are most often established with private practices in the area. This can be seen as a positive move for the private practice, because it brings them in as part of an alliance with a larger health care system. It also provides those physical therapists working in private practice the flexibility of working for a private practice and a hospital (through contract) and enjoying the perks of a higher salary and other benefits offered by the private practice. Physical therapists will always be needed in the acute care setting regardless of their employment status (salaried or on contract).

DIRECT ACCESS   ### Background

Historically, the Reconstruction Aide worked closely with the physician, carrying out orders for exercise, massage or therapeutic modalities to be applied to the patient. Prescriptions were written by the physician which specified the type of exercise to be performed, modality to be used, and intensity and duration of the treatment. As the education of the physical therapist expanded, so too did the knowledge base and hands-on skills. However, as noted above, the educational programs, under the auspices of the AMA, were never updated or revised until 1955.

As the educational preparation of the physical therapist expanded after 1955, the provision of physical therapy to the consumer changed as well. In 1957, Nebraska became the first state to have direct access. This enabled the citizens of Nebraska to obtain treatment from a physical therapist without seeing a physician first and being referred to the therapist. The second state to enact legislation for direct access was California in 1968. Legislation proliferated in the 1980s and early 1990s to enable physical therapists to practice with direct access. In the states that allow direct access, physical therapists evaluate the patient, determine an appropriate treatment and render that treatment based on their findings.

Direct Access Today

There are now 30 states in the country that enable the physical therapist to practice with direct access. The concept behind direct access is to enable the consumer to have the choice of accessing the physical therapist or the physician. If the physical therapist determines that the patient's problem is outside of her/his scope of practice, or needs further medical assessment, the patient is referred to the primary care physician. Providing the consumer direct access to the physical therapist contributes to the reduction of health care costs (by eliminating the physician office visit to obtain the referral), and expedites initiation of appropriate treatment. In states without direct access, patients may wait four to six weeks to see the physician, only to have the physician write a referral for physical therapy without a comprehensive evaluation, and then charging for a full office visit. Upon seeing the physical therapist (4–6 weeks post injury) the acute problem may now have developed into a chronic problem with additional secondary problems (such as protective muscle spasms and contracture).

Direct access has worked effectively in those states in which it has been adopted. In those states without such legislation, resistance to direct access has been primarily from the physician's professional organization. Concerns have been raised that physical therapists do not have enough knowledge to diagnose problems that the patient presents, and as a result, malpractice suits will result.

In reality, malpractice suits have not increased in those states with direct access. Moreover, in states without direct access, a diagnosis is not typically noted on the physician's referral. The majority of patients referred to physical therapy from a physician have on the referral "Evaluate and Treat" or a symptom such as low back pain or knee pain. Neither of these are diagnoses which would aid the physical therapist in determining a treatment plan. The treatment plan for the patient is developed after the physical therapist completes the evaluation.

The other unspoken concern of the physician's professional organization is that the number of patients in their care will be reduced if the physical therapist has direct access. This has not been documented as a problem, or reality, in any of the states with direct access.

The Future of Direct Access with Health Care Reform

The key to direct access with health care reform will be the establishment of the **"gate-keepers"** or "gateways" into the health care system. Historically, the primary care physician has been the access (gatekeeper) into the health care system. It is the primary care physician who then refers patients to physical therapists, physician specialists, or other health care providers. The limited number of physicians entering the field of primary health care has opened the door for the nurse practitioner and the physician's assistant to serve as the entry point into health care especially in the rural settings. Some of the proposed federal legislation would enable any licensed health care provider practicing within the individual's scope of practice to be an entry point for the consumer into health care. If this type of legislation is passed, it would enable the consumer in any state to have direct access to physical therapy care.

The APTA has provided testimony for the establishment of physical therapists as one of the "gateways" into the health care system, citing the education, knowledge, and skill level of the physical therapist as evidence of ability to serve as an entry point into health care.

PHYSICIAN-OWNED PHYSICAL THERAPY SERVICES

As previously noted, the physician has been the primary coordinator of the treatment that a patient receives. The physician orders the necessary diagnostic work, requests consults from other health care providers and orders the treatment regimen for the patient. With this responsibility and control, many physicians have established clinics where they own all of the diagnostic equipment, laboratory equipment, pharmacies, and physical therapy clinics. The physicians refer their patients to their own clinics. When this occurs, the patient has lost the choice of where to go for diagnostic work or treatment, and the potential for overuse of the services is created.

A **physician-owned physical therapy service (POPTS)** is an example of the overuse that can occur when a physician has a financial investment in a clinic. Two studies conducted in Florida and California have demonstrated that when the physician has ownership in physical therapy services, there is an overuse of the physical therapy care resulting in overspending of health care dollars.[6, 11] These two studies have shown that when physicians have ownership in a physical therapy clinic, they continue to refer patients for physical therapy care even when the patient has plateaued or reached established goals. Patients have also been *inappropriately* referred and treated in such clinical settings.

The American Medical Association reported in the American Medical News that it is unethical for a physician to have a financial investment in a lab or clinic to which he or she refers.[5] Federal legislation (the Stark Law) has been enacted to prohibit patients on Medicare from receiving care in a lab or clinic in which the referring physician or a family member owns an interest. A related law effective January 1, 1995, expanded this limitation to Medicaid patients as well.

To avoid the unethical and potentially illegal situation of owning an interest in a physical therapy clinic, many physicians hire physical therapists to work as their employees. The same abuse of overutilization of physical therapy care can and does exist in this environment, but employment of a physical therapist to work in the physician's office is currently not restricted in any way.

ENCROACHMENT AND HUMAN RESOURCES

Encroachment is defined in *Webster's Dictionary* as
1. to trespass or intrude (on or upon the rights, property, etc. of another); 2. to advance beyond the proper, original, or customary limits."[12]

In the health care arena, encroachment occurs when one health care provider performs the skills and techniques of another health care provider.

Physical therapy is provided by physical therapists and physical therapist assistants. In some states, the physical therapy aide, a layperson trained by the PT, can also provide limited physical therapy treatment in a physical therapy clinic. But the problem of the inadequate supply of physical therapists and physical therapist assistants does not meet the consumer demand.

In the absence of qualified physical therapy professionals to meet the demands of the consumer, other health care providers fill the void. This occurs most often with athletic trainers and occupational therapists. An example is the rehabilitation of the week-end athlete. If an individual injures his/her knee in a basketball game and develops edema (swelling), pain, and restricted mobility, that person should be treated by a physical therapist. Since the injury occurred in a sporting event, the athletic trainer might say that the individual should be treated by an athletic trainer. Who is encroaching on the other's territory? Both providers should not be providing the same treatment to the patient and receiving reimbursement.

In another example, a physical therapist and occupational therapist (OT) are treating an individual who had a stroke and are instructing the patient in bathtub transfers. This is a duplication of services for which both units are receiving reimbursement. Who is encroaching on the other health care professional's territory?

These types of questions are being raised all over the country as each health care profession strives to maintain its own identity and professional integrity. The answers to some of these questions may differ depending on the different practice acts which regulate and govern health care professionals in each state. In New York State, for example, the physical therapist would be responsible for the acute rehabilitation of the week-end athlete's knee injury. However, either the athletic trainer or the physical therapist could recondition the individual for return to recreational activities. The treatment provided by the physical therapist would be reimbursed as physical therapy. The treatment provided by the athletic trainer is not reimbursable, as there are no billing codes to cover athletic training care, and it is illegal for a trainer to bill for physical therapy, unless that person is a licensed physical therapist. This is further explained in the section on Reimbursement.

The bathtub transfer scenario could be performed by both the OT and PT as long as they are both working on different outcomes for the patient. For example, the PT may be doing the transfer activity for the sole purpose of enabling the patient to be independent in the transfer. The occupational therapy goal would be more global, incorporating the activity of daily care: the patient will be independent in bathing in the bathtub. To accomplish this goal, the patient must be able to perform the transfer as well as manage bathing activities in the tub.

Human Resources

The biggest factor contributing to encroachment in different health care professions is the shortage of professionally trained personnel that may exist in a profession and the resulting inability of that profession to meet the service demands of the public. There has been a critical shortage of physical therapists for at least a decade, even though there has been a proliferation in the number of schools graduating physical therapists. In 1992, physical therapy schools graduated 4850 new therapists, but 7000 vacancies still remained.[10] In June 1994, the APTA reported that there were 85,000 physical therapists in the United States, of which 2 percent were retired or not working. This leaves approximately 83,300 physical therapists to fill 90,000 physical therapy jobs. A growth of 88 percent is expected in physical therapy by 2005 according to the U.S. Department of Labor. Projections indicate that most professions will grow by 22 percent during that time frame.[4]

Enrolling and graduating more physical therapists could be an answer to this problem; however, the shortage of physical therapy faculty is already straining the existing programs. A survey conducted by the APTA in 1991 of the physical therapist education programs indicated that 78 faculty vacancies existed in bachelor's degree programs and 45 faculty vacancies existed in postbaccalaureate programs.[9] The vacancy rate includes faculty, academic coordinators of clinical education and academic administrators, and is based on an 82 percent response rate to the survey. Of the 772 faculty included in the survey, 42 percent held a doctorate. As physical therapy education moves further into postbaccalaureate education, the majority of physical therapy faculty will be required to have a doctorate to remain employable in an academic institution. The limited number of faculty in physical therapist education programs with a doctorate further contributes to the faculty shortage.

REIMBURSEMENT

One of the major issues fueling the health care reform debate is this: Who is going to pay for the health care needed by the employed and unemployed in this country? Our current health care system is based on **reimbursement** for health care services through health insurance obtained through an employer, private insurance, Medicare, or Medicaid. A physical therapist providing physical therapy care to a patient uses billing codes that are appropriate for the type of treatment provided to the patient. The bill is then sent to the insurance company for reimbursement. The billing codes used for physical therapy services are not exclusive to physical therapists. These same billing codes are used by physicians and podiatrists. Monitoring overutilization of these billing codes is difficult, because so many different health care providers use the codes.

With inequities in reimbursement and overutilization of health care services, health care costs have been skyrocketing. Reimbursement for a billing code is different for a physician and a physical therapist. If a physical therapist applies a hot pack to a patient, the PT will be reimbursed a certain amount, but if the physician applies the hot pack in the office, he/she is often reimbursed ten times what the PT receives. The application of the hot pack is the same, the physiologic effects of heat are the same, but the physician is reimbursed more for the treatment provided.

Development of physical therapy specific billing codes is one way to address the reimbursement problem for physical therapists. Establishment of nation-wide billing codes exclusive to physical therapists would enable the formation of physical therapy peer review panels to regulate the delivery of physical therapy care. Physical therapy specific billing codes would also prevent the physical therapy allotment in an individual's insurance plan from being exhausted by any other health professional using the same billing codes. For example, if a patient receives a whirlpool treatment at a podiatrist's office, the cost of that whirlpool treatment is often logged against the available insurance plan dollars for physical therapy reimbursement provided by a physical therapist. The result is fewer dollars available for physical therapy services provided by a PT.

The regulations that are in place to monitor the cost, quality, and utilization of the health care services by the patient and the health care professional are not adequate to control the system. Tighter restrictions must be developed to insure that the consumer is receiving quality care and at a reasonable cost.

Reform of the reimbursement system must occur, the question is how soon and to what extent. The issues described here are only a few of the many reimbursement problems that face physical therapists. Physical therapists practicing in institutions such as hospitals and rehabilitation centers have previously been protected from these reimbursement problems; the private practice was the setting that was affected the most. Currently, hospital physical therapy operating budgets are being cut, and vacant physical therapist positions are not being filled in order to decrease costs due to lack of reimbursement. The result is that reimbursement problems affect both the consumer and the provider.

CONTINUOUS QUALITY IMPROVEMENT

Continuous Quality Improvement or Total Quality Management (CQI/TQM) is "a method of examining and improving processes using data management tools."[13] Simply put it means using data that are collected every day to improve the quality of a service that is provided. It has been a component of most hospitals for several years and has also been integrated into most physical therapy practice settings. Total Quality Management in a physical therapy clinic would consist of continual assessment on how physical therapy care is being delivered and on the patient outcome. In the early implementation of TQM, physical therapists would document the number of patient visits, cancellations, and no-shows. Now it has expanded to consider how efficiently the care is delivered, and if the patient achieves the desired outcome.

As TQM has developed in hospitals, it has led to the advent of a new patient delivery model called **patient-focused care (PFC).** In this model, all departments in a hospital are decentralized, and professional staff are assigned to work on multi-disciplinary teams. Instead of the PT department being located on one floor, and all the patients being transported to PT, the therapist is now stationed on a nursing unit with other health care providers to provide treatment to a core group of patients with similar problems. A good example of this is the physical therapist working on a multi-disciplinary team for orthopaedic surgical patients. All members of the team are on the floor with the patients and all services that the patients need are brought to them. This has decreased the wasted time that health care providers spend trying to find a patient because the individual left the nursing floor for tests or other reasons. The team coordinates the treatment to be provided to each patient at the beginning of every day, and there are shared responsibilities among members of the team. Trained technicians are part of the team to carry out much of the basic care for the patient preceded by instruction from the physical therapist. This may include transfers of the patient and ambulation.

The patient-focused care model has also brought with it the controversy of **cross-training** of health care professionals. This has sent a shock wave through most of the physical therapy professional community. Cross-training could include physical therapists doing some physical therapy care, occupational therapy care, and nursing care for the patient. The concept of cross-training originally grew out of the inadequate supply of physical therapists available to work in the hospitals; therefore, training occupational therapists and nurses to perform some of the physical therapy services was a necessity. In addition, cross-training not only affects physical therapy, but all health care professions. Treatment skills from a variety of professions would be integrated to be provided by members of a multi-disciplinary team.

The PFC model does introduce some cross-training of the members of the multi-disciplinary team, but many physical therapists working in this model state that the important evaluative and treatment components of physical therapy have been retained by the physical therapist. In many settings, therapists report that members of the multi-disciplinary team have a better understanding and appreciation for the knowledge base of the physical therapist.

A very positive development of the PFC model is the development of **critical pathways,** which are defined by Woods as "a guideline for patient care during hospital stay using 'milestones' to progress patient; a guide based on consensus, including only those aspects of care provided to affect patient outcomes."[13] The critical pathway is a planned sequence of treatment progression based on the patient's response and recovery. Initiating physical therapy treatment is an established part of the critical pathway, so a delay in receiving physician's orders does not occur. Likewise, the physical therapy progression of the patient is also a component of the pathway. Some therapists who use the system report that the critical pathways are clearly defining the parameters of our practice and the role that the physical therapist should play in the rehabilitation of the patient.

RESEARCH IN
PHYSICAL
THERAPY

To address many of the issues that have been discussed in this chapter, evidence is needed to support the effectiveness of physical therapy care. Demonstrating improved patient outcomes as a result of physical therapy intervention will ensure the identity and integrity of our profession. Physical therapy is an art and a science, but clinical based research is needed to substantiate the science component of the profession.

The major emphasis of physical therapy research must be in two areas: (1) the establishment of measurement tools that are valid, reliable and measure patient outcomes; and (2) the efficacy of physical therapy treatment.[8] The best environment for investigation of these areas is in the physical therapy clinic. The Research Center established by the Foundation for Physical Therapy is an excellent example of advancing research in measurement and treatment efficacy. The University of Iowa was awarded a three-year grant from the Foundation to establish a research center focusing on total hip and knee replacements and ultrasound treatment. The Foundation hopes to fund three other such centers in the country with emphasis on the following: low back injury and carpal tunnel syndrome, sports and catastrophe-related injuries, and treatment of older persons (see Chapter 4). This type of focused research is needed to demonstrate the role that physical therapy plays in prevention and rehabilitation.

Clinicians who work with patients every day are another source of data collection for studying treatment outcomes. Unfortunately, the majority of practicing physical therapists have limited experience in research methodology. A stronger collaboration of physical therapy faculty with clinicians must be developed to facilitate clinical based research. Another means to address this is to foster students in post-professional physical therapy education programs to carry out clinical based research in conjunction with clinicians.

SUMMARY

This chapter reviewed the current issues affecting physical therapy. Educational preparation of the physical therapist remains an issue to be debated on the floor of the House of Delegates as the profession moves toward the DPT degree. The role of the physical therapist assistant is expanding from that of a technician to a para-professional. The practice settings may change with the advent of health care reform. Physical therapists and PTAs will continue to work in the hospitals, but the status of private practice as we know it today may quickly change with managed care. Legislation for direct access may become obsolete if health care reform enables the consumer to access any health care provider practicing within the individual's scope of practice. Any physician-owned physical therapy practice should become illegal with the enactment of federal legislation. Encroachment will continue until there are an adequate number of health care providers in each field to meet the consumers' demands.

All of these issues, however, will not be resolved on their own. Resolution of most will require the active participation of physical therapists and physical therapist assistants in the local, state, and national levels of the APTA. Interactions with other members of the health care team will also be necessary to address common issues that face everyone affected by health care reform.

References

1. 1993 Active membership profile report, Alexandria, VA, 1994, American Physical Therapy Association.

2. American Hospital Association. One North Franklin, Chicago, personal communication.

3. Entry-level education, HOD 06-80-10-29, Alexandria, VA, 1979, American Physical Therapy Association.

4. Growth of physical therapy to continue into next century, PT Bulletin 9(18):2, May 11, 1994.

5. HCFA weighs option for wider referral ban, American Medical News 37(23):1, June 20, 1994.

6. Joint ventures among health care providers in Florida, State of Florida, conducted by Florida Health Care Cost Containment Board in conjunction with Dept of Economics and Dept of Finance, Florida State Univ. August 1991.

7. Managed care, managed fair, American Medical News 37(19):13, Aug 1, 1994.

8. Model for targeting research areas in physical therapy, Alexandria, VA, 1994, American Physical Therapy Association.

9. Physical therapist education programs, Alexandria, VA, 1992, American Physical Therapy Association.

10. Pinkston D: Evolution of the practice of physical therapy in the United States. In Scully RM, Barnes MR, editors: Physical Therapy, Philadelphia, 1989, JB Lippincott Company.

11. Swedlow A, et al: Increased costs and rates of use in the California worker's compensation system as a result of self-referral by physicians, N Eng J Med 327(21):1502-1506, November, 1992.

12. Webster's New World Dictionary, Second College Edition. Simon and Schuster, New York, NY 1986.

13. Woods EN: The restructuring of America's hospitals: what does it mean for physical therapy? PT-Magazine of Phys Ther 2(6):34-41, 1994.

Suggested Readings

PT Bulletin, Alexandria, VA, American Physical Therapy Association. Contains short articles and letters to the editor which address current issues. Published weekly and distributed to all members of the APTA.

House of Delegates policies, Alexandria, VA, American Physical Therapy Association. Updated annually including new goals for the APTA.

PT-Magazine of Physical Therapy, Alexandria, VA, American Physical Therapy Association. May issue of this monthly publication distributed to members of APTA includes the Annual Report of the APTA.

Stewart D and Abeln S: Documenting Functional Outcomes in Physical Therapy, St. Louis, MO, 1993, Mosby-Year Book. This text discusses a variety of documentation models that demonstrate the conceptual framework of clinical decision analysis. Examples of appropriate and inappropriate reporting are given along with the expectations of a variety of payers. Case studies are included.

Depoy E and Gitlin S: Introduction to Research: Multiple Strategies for Health and Human Services, St. Louis, MO, 1993, Mosby-Year Book. This introductory text was written for members of all allied health professions and teaches the reader how to critically evaluate, implement, and respect a variety of research strategies.

Review Questions

1. Explain the controversy over consideration of a DPT program. What issues does it raise?

2. Discuss both sides of the debate over PTA attendance at continuing education PT courses.

3. Why is it more difficult for PTs than physicians to establish a contractual relationship with an HMO?

4. Weigh the objections to direct access against its track record in states that legislate in its favor.

5. Explain the risks involved in a POPTS.

6. What is "encroachment"? Discuss the issues it raises and their impact on reimbursement for services.

7. Explain the advantages of developing physical therapy specific billing codes, both from the PT and consumer perspectives. Do you see any drawbacks?

8. Give balanced attention to analyzing the advantages and disadvantages seen in the patient-focused care model.

Part II
Practice

Chapter 7

Pediatric Physical Therapy

Angela M. Easley

"What path will we take? Let us not take one that others have made... Instead, let us make our own path."
Ruth Wood, PT, FAPTA

KEY TERMS

assessment process
cerebral palsy (CP)
clubfoot
conductive education
congenital dislocation of the hip (CDH)
continuum of disablement
cystic fibrosis (CF)
developmental delays (DD)
disability
Downs syndrome
Duchenne muscular dystrophy (DMD)
eclectic approach
evaluation
family assessment
fetal alcohol syndrome (FAS)
handicap

impairment
individualized education plan (IEP)
individualized family services plan (IFSP)
juvenile rheumatoid arthritis (JRA)
meningocele
meningomyelocele
neurodevelopmental treatment approach (NDT)
normal developmental theory
objective examination
osteogenesis imperfecta (OI)
prenatal cocaine exposure
scoliosis
screening
sensory integration theory (SI)
spina bifida
spina bifida occulta
spinal muscular atrophy (SMA)
standardized testing
subjective examination

Children will be children first and foremost. They are not merely scaled-down versions of adults, rather they progress through unique age-related movement stages, or milestones. Pediatric physical therapists will assess these milestones to determine if discrepancies exist between the child's chronological and neurological (or developmental) ages. If so, evaluation and subsequent treatment may be appropriate. This chapter describes the evaluation and treatment techniques used by the pediatric physical therapist. It includes common conditions seen and two case studies to illustrate a variety of approaches for the management of pediatric clients.

GENERAL
DESCRIPTION

The primary focus for pediatric therapists, is to observe children as they portray their individual strengths and abilities and to promote a functional, quality developmental process. By acquiring knowledge of normal development through observation of movement patterns and transitions, abnormal movements can be more accurately detected. The challenge is determining normal delays from those that signal potential developmental problems.[22] For example, observations of generations of children tell us that walking is initiated at approximately 10 to 13 months, yet some infants may take their first steps as early as 8 months, or as late as 18 months! This type of variation occurs at all stages of child development and requires pediatric therapists to evaluate and treat children on a constantly changing developmental base.[17]

In addition to child development, pediatric practice requires the therapist to acquire a specific knowledge in basic areas ranging from child psychology to motor learning. The cognitive strategies and learning methods of adults are generally functionally oriented toward work, leisure or daily living activities, while children learn from a different point of view—play. The pediatric physical therapist is often found in what might be called compromising situations—hopping, rolling, tumbling—in order to engage the child and invite him or her to participate in therapeutic activities.

Play is the medium most utilized to promote therapeutic activities for the young child, while for the adolescent, therapy goals may be structured around social situations.[49] The primary goal is to identify meaningful activities which correspond to the learning style of each pediatric client, given the age, culture and most natural social and physical environments (Fig. 7-1).

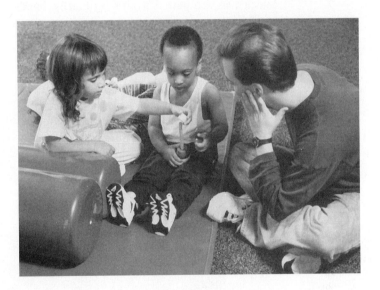

Fig. 7-1. Cooperative play is a primary base for therapeutic activities (Photo credit: Bruce Wang).

Children who have health problems that require specialty or subspecialty care are referred to as "children with special health care needs."[75] Pediatric therapists often provide therapy to these children over long periods of time. When caring for children with special needs, physical therapists collaborate closely with the family and other health professionals in designing a long-term, family-centered plan of care. This plan includes a full range of services—prevention, early identification, evaluation, diagnostics, treatment, habilitation, and rehabilitation.[56] Throughout service provision, the emphasis is placed on recognizing each child as part of a family system, with unique cultural characteristics that must be considered when designing treatment goals.

If the physical therapist focuses solely on the child's motor strengths and needs, while neglecting the cultural impact of family and community factors on that child, a successful treatment outcome is unlikely (Fig. 7-2). The World Health Organization (WHO) recognized this focus by viewing a **continuum of disablement** on several levels: impairment, disability and handicap, acknowledging their inter-relationship and impact on one another (Table 7-1).[37,47] Through this model, it becomes evident that physical **impairment** (e.g., central nervous system abnormality) directly affects the child in several realms, including the physical, all of which must be considered when designing a plan of care. The child's **disability** or the manifestation of the impairment (e.g., inability to speak or walk) is influenced by the family system (e.g., interaction style) and also will have an impact on family interactions and peer relationships. Finally, **handicap,** the influence of social/environmental factors on disability (e.g., access to schools, sports) is a result of the culture, society and environment in which the child lives.

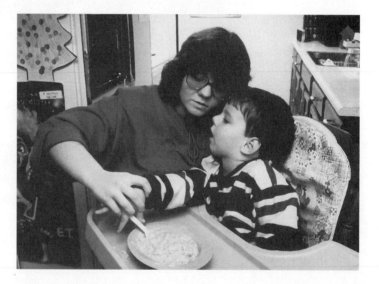

Fig. 7-2. A mother assisting her son's special motor needs at dinner time (Photo credit: Bruce Wang).

Table 7-1: Classification of Disablement*

Disablement Classification	Characteristics	Interaction Level
Impairment	Physical Cognitive Perceptual Communication Social	Child
Disability	Urban/Rural Interaction Style Relationships	Family
Handicap	Economy Public Policy Religion Health Care System Architecture	Community

* Adapted from International Classification of Impairment, Disability and Handicap, Geneva, Switzerland, 1980, World Health Organization.

When the child is cared for using this model as a guide, all of these factors are considered as equal elements in designing a plan of care. In addition, it is important to note in the WHO classification that these disablement categories are not mutually exclusive. A child's physical condition can influence and be influenced by her/his cognitive awareness, social interactions, and community practices. In a climate of radical health care reform and shifting venues for pediatric practice, a practitioner's understanding of the interdependence of all levels is germane to treatment success.

Impact of Federal Legislation

The scope of pediatric specialization within the field of physical therapy is rapidly evolving due to a variety of factors which directly affect the care of children: public policy, family-centered care, and environments for practice. These elements, although seemingly unrelated, have become entwined through the passage of federal legislation unique to the practice of pediatrics.

The Education for All Handicapped Children's Act (EHCA), Public Law 94-142, passed in 1975, was landmark legislation that has continued to shape and evolve the nature of pediatric practice for all professional disciplines.[28] The main premise of the EHCA was that all children from ages 6 to 21 years, regardless of disability, were entitled to free and appropriate public education. This premise set the basic framework for policy and standards which were amended in 1986 with the passage of Public Law 99-457 (Amendments to the EHCA) and again in 1991, with re-authorization as the Individuals with Disabilities Education Act (IDEA).[46] These amendments provide distinct policy for children from birth through two, and three through five years of age. Embedded within the amendments is specific language which stipulates the concept of parent/professional collaboration and a family-centered focus throughout the process of pediatric assessment, intervention, and care coordination. In addition, this legislation set forth policy guidelines that require that children be cared for in their "least restrictive" or "natural environments" ranging from home to day care centers as optimal sites for physical therapy intervention (Fig. 7-3 A and B).[46]

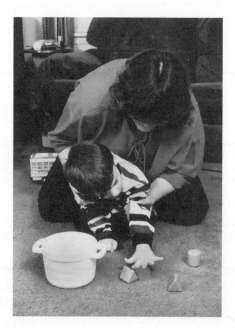 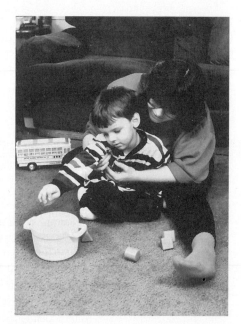

Fig. 7-3 A,B. Therapy at home—a natural environment (Photo credits: Bruce Wang).

The focus on the family system, family-centered care, individualized child and family plans, and natural environments is now commonplace in pediatric practice. This focus on family, in essence, speaks to the evolving societal and cultural contexts in which pediatric physical therapists collaborate in the care of children with special needs.

COMMON
CONDITIONS

It is impractical to list the full range of pediatric diagnostic conditions in this chapter. Children, like adults, have conditions which require expertise in all specialty areas. Many children are seen for acute, short-term orthopaedic needs, such as the child who sprains her ankle while playing soccer. The majority of these pediatric clients are seen in physical therapy outpatient orthopaedic clinics or by sports physical therapy specialists.

Another subset of pediatric clients, and the group most associated with pediatric practice are children diagnosed with **developmental delays (DD)** and disabilities. A child with a developmental delay has not attained predictable movement patterns or behaviors that are associated with children of a similar chronological age. In the course of fetal developmental, there are a multitude of risk factors that have the potential to cause a developmental problem. These factors, such as genetic and chromosomal anomalies or environmental toxins, may cause impairment to the central or peripheral nervous system resulting in immediate or eventual developmental delays or potential disability. These children generally require some combination of short- and long-term therapies which continually shift given each child's changing physical, cognitive, and emotional abilities.

The remainder of this section consists of brief descriptions of selected pediatric conditions which are categorized as orthopaedic, genetic, or environmental in nature. Later in the chapter, two of these conditions will be described through vignettes of children to provide the reader with snapshots of the many "faces" of pediatric practice.

Orthopaedic Disorders

Children may be born with or acquire problems with bones, muscles, fascia, and joints. Some of the more common disorders are discussed below.

Juvenile Rheumatoid Arthritis (JRA). One of the many rheumatic diseases, juvenile rheumatoid arthritis is characterized by an inflammation of the connective tissue which manifests as a painful inflamed joint (arthritis). The actual cause of JRA is unknown with possibilities ranging from a viral onset to genetic predisposition.[20,69] Juvenile rheumatoid arthritis may manifest in several distinct forms or subtypes each with different characteristics. These subtypes vary in the number of joints affected, age of onset, male:female ratio, clinical findings, and prognosis. Signs and symptoms usually include joint pain, swelling, decreased motion, stiffness, and muscle atrophy. The majority of children diagnosed with JRA lead active lives, with the assistance of medications, therapeutic exercise assistance, and specialized care programs. It is generally believed that an interdisciplinary team including parents, a pediatric rheumatologist, nurse, psychologist, physical therapist, and occupational therapist is best for total care coordination.

The primary role of the physical therapist is to assist in the prevention of deformity and improvement of the overall quality of life for the child. A primary focus is generally the musculoskeletal needs of the child with a special emphasis on those needs which affect function. Individualized goals are collaboratively formed to address posture, strength, mobility, and joint motion within the child's daily functional routine. Parent and child collaboration, education, and instruction are vital as the home is where the majority of the child's goals will be reinforced.[69]

Clubfoot. The name is derived from the position of the afflicted foot, which is turned inward and slanted upward. Because of this position, certain muscles become shortened, causing the foot to remain in a fixed position. Treatment includes progressive and prolonged casting, as well as manual correction immediately after birth.

Scoliosis. Scoliosis is characterized by a lateral curvature of the spine. The curve may vary in severity from mild to severe. Scoliosis may be idiopathic (unknown origin), neuromuscular, or congenital (present at birth). Scoliosis is now detected more frequently due to school-based screening programs and is noted by asymmetries of the shoulders, breasts, and pelvis among other factors. Treatment involves a wide range of external or internal fixations, and in select cases, electrical stimulation, depending on the degree of development of the curve. Exercise assists in reducing back pain and improving range of motion.

Congenital Dislocation of the Hip (CDH). This results from the abnormal development of some of the structures surrounding the hip joint allowing the head of the femur (thigh bone) to move in and out of the hip socket. The cause is unknown, but thought to be related to a number of factors such as maternal hormonal changes during pregnancy, birth trauma, or improper positioning after birth. Treatment involves manually or surgically returning the femoral head to the hip socket and stabilizing it with splints or casts, depending on the degree of impairment and age of the child. Intensive exercise protocols are required post-surgically to regain range of joint motion, muscle strength, and function. Children with spina bifida and certain forms of cerebral palsy are more prone to congenital dislocation of the hip and are monitored through regular physical examinations.

Osteogenesis Imperfecta (OI). This is a common and severe bone impairment of genetic origin. The genetic defect affects the formation of collagen during bone development resulting in frequent fractures during the fetal or newborn period. The fetal form of OI is associated with high mortality, while the infantile form is less severe, with increased vulnerability for frequent fractures of the long bones in early childhood. Children with OI are identified through characteristic limb deformities, dental abnormalities, stunted growth, scoliosis, loose ligaments, and an unusually shaped skull. Treatment of fractures and prevention of deformity are the major focus of treatment, as well as gentle exercise after post-surgical healing has occurred.

Genetic Disorders

Duchenne Muscular Dystrophy (DMD). With this disorder, females do not manifest symptoms but become carriers of the disease; whereas males do manifest symptoms. Boys with Duchenne muscular dystrophy usually develop normally until 6 to 9 years of age, when progressive pelvic muscle weakness and wasting becomes apparent and are combined with enlarged, yet weak, thigh muscles and tight heel cords. Associated complications include muscle contractures, spinal curvature (scoliosis), and wheelchair dependence at 10 to 12 years of age. Progressive weakness, pneumonia, and cardiac abnormalities eventually reduce the lifespan of persons with DMD.[8] Developmentally, the child with Duchenne muscular dystrophy may present with mild mental retardation or learning disabilities, low muscle tone, and delays in attainment of motor milestones.[45]

Spinal Muscular Atrophy (SMA). Symptoms of this disorder include severe muscle weakness in infancy and progressive respiratory failure. Developmentally, children with SMA in the infantile form have a decreased life span, whereas children with the juvenile form have increased survival but require aggressive physical therapy and orthopaedic management.[76]

Spina bifida. Spina bifida is a prenatal disorder involving orthopaedic malformations in its mild form and neurological malformations in its severe form (Fig. 7-4). Although the etiology is unknown, the neurological impairment appears to be a result of faulty closure of the neural groove in the first month of pregnancy. Recent hypotheses suggest that this impairment may be a result of genetic expression in combination with factors in the fetal (maternal) environment.[50] Environmental factors such as organic solvents, ethanol and valproic acid have been suggested, and most recently maternal folate deficiency appears to exert a strong influence.[48,53,55]

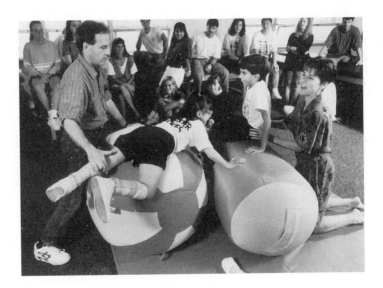

Fig. 7-4. Physical therapists promote interactive play to assist the movement patterns of two children diagnosed with spina bifida (Photo credit: Bruce Wang).

Below are several types of neural tube defects that differ in level of severity depending on the degree of vertebral closure and spinal cord exposure:

Spina Bifida Occulta. A common impairment of a vertebra (separation of the spinous process) that is not associated with disability and may only be discovered through diagnostic tests such as radiographic studies.

Meningocele. A benign herniation of the meninges presenting as a soft tissue cyst or lump that surrounds a normal spinal cord resulting in no neurological deficits.

Meningomyelocele. An open lesion with minimal to no skin protection containing the deeper nerve roots. This condition is the most severe with the potential for leakage of spinal fluid, and infection prior to surgical intervention and healing. Because this impairment is usually at the lower end of the spine, there is often resultant loss of motor function and sensation of the lower body including problems with bowel and bladder function.

Chromosomal Disorders

Cystic Fibrosis (CF). This pulmonary disorder is the most common inherited chronic disease among Caucasian children. It is characterized by the production of thick mucus with progressive lung damage. Children with CF require frequent hospitalizations due to acute respiratory attacks. There are a variety of medications and therapies that assist in decreasing the side effects of this disease as well as genetic research, which has resulted in recent isolation of the defective gene.[64]

Downs syndrome. **Downs syndrome** is a congenital developmental disability caused by a defect of the 21st chromosome; it is sometimes called Trisomy 21. The child with Downs syndrome is characterized by low muscle tone, a flat facial profile, upwardly slanted eyes, short stature, mental retardation, slowed growth and development, a small nose with a low nasal bridge, and congenital heart disease.[7,63,71] Associated complications may include instability of the first and second vertebrae, lax ligaments, seizures, leukemia, and premature senility.[2,6,62] The combination of these features often manifest in deficiencies in balance, stability, and agility across many tasks and environmental contexts. Developmentally, the child with Downs syndrome has decreased muscle tone which improves with age. This is offset by the loose ligaments that result in increased range of joint   otion. The level of mental retardation varies with the rate of developmental progress decreasing with age.[24,62]

Environmentally Related Disorders

A variety of risk factors affecting either the health of the mother or fetus may present a risk to the newborn infant's health. Some of these factors include maternal health and nutrition (e.g., vitamin deficiency), radiation, drugs, infections, environmental toxins (e.g., lead), pre- or post-labor infant hypoxia (lack of oxygen), and birth trauma. Depending on the nature of and timing of the presentation of the risk factor during the pregnancy, the newborn may present with a variety of developmental disabilities ranging from mild to severe in nature.

Cerebral Palsy (CP). This is a group of conditions, rather than a disease, caused by a non-progressive lesion on the brain. Most often CP occurs during gestation (before birth), at birth, or immediately after birth due to an interruption of oxygen to the brain of the fetus or newborn.[65] A variety of environmental toxins, maternal or infant infections, or an early childhood trauma can cause this condition. The core problem with cerebral palsy is the inability of the brain to control nerve and muscle activity. The manifestation of cerebral palsy differs depending on the cause, timing (age of fetus/child), and location and extent of the original impairment to the brain. Often early signs of cerebral palsy include poor sucking, irritability, stiff muscles (hypertonia), or floppy muscles (hypotonia). Later manifestations may include delayed motor milestones, poor coordination, involuntary movements (dyskinesia), writhing movements (athetosis), poor visual tracking (ability of the eyes to follow a moving object), and language delays.[1] Approximately 60 percent to 70 percent of all children with CP are mentally retarded.[10] Management emphasis is on attaining optimal growth and development. A variety of specialists may be involved in caring for the child with CP including physical therapists, occupational therapists, and speech and language pathologists. In many cases, neurosurgical intervention, orthotics, adaptive equipment, or pharmacological intervention is required to ameliorate or correct deformities (Fig. 7-5).[73]

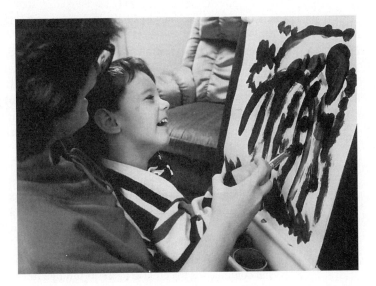

Fig. 7-5. All smiles when painting is a part of therapy for a child with cerebral palsy (Photo credit: Bruce Wang).

Fetal Alcohol Syndrome (FAS). This is the most severe condition in a continuum of alcohol-induced disabilities.[52] It is related to high levels of maternal alcohol consumption during pregnancy. **Fetal Alcohol Syndrome (FAS)** is the leading known cause of mental retardation, surpassing Downs syndrome and spina bifida. Children are generally born at term (on their due date) but are smaller than normal weight and height. Children with FAS have distinct physical features that assist in identifying them with FAS. Complications are widespread and include an increased incidence of congenital heart defects, joint contractures, visual and auditory impairments and hip dislocation.[36] Developmentally, the child with FAS may experience a range of delays in the areas of language, fine motor control, eye-hand coordination, speech, IQ, and psycho-social behaviors.[72]

Prenatal Cocaine Exposure. This disorder is related to fetal exposure to cocaine in utero due to maternal cocaine use during pregnancy.[21,68] Infants often present with clinical signs of exposure after birth including hyperirritability, poor feeding patterns, high respiratory and heart rates, increased tremulousness, and irregular sleeping patterns.[57] Developmentally, the child exposed to cocaine may experience abnormalities in muscle tone, reflexes, movement, and attention which may continue many months after birth.[27,67] If these problems persist, including increased muscle tone or tremors, other developmental milestones may be delayed.[66] Research studies regarding the long-term effects of fetal cocaine exposure are currently being conducted nationwide.

EVALUATION
PRINCIPLES AND
TECHNIQUES

The screening, evaluation, and assessment of children involves measures to determine if a child is in need of physical therapy intervention as well as to monitor the child's progress after physical therapy has been initiated. If a child is suspected of having or is at risk for a developmental disability, an **assessment process** is initiated which involves close monitoring, evaluation and, if indicated, initiation of treatment. This process is ongoing and involves many subjective and objective measurements that describe the child's initial and ongoing progress.

A combination of subjective and objective information about a child is generally obtained through discussions with family members and, if possible, with the child. For a child up to three years of age, the **subjective examination** of the care plan may take the form of a family assessment.[5] Family assessment is an essential part of the plan because the child will be treated in the context of his/her family system. The **family assessment** is defined as a process that begins with the referral of a child for services and continues as the child progresses through the various parts of the pediatric system.[30] Family assessment may take the form of an interview, discussion, or standardized survey and is often initiated by the team member who will be the primary coordinator of care for the family. Regardless of the format, the purpose of family assessment is to gain the family's insights regarding the child, including family history, relationships, satisfactions, concerns, needs, and resources. This information has direct impact on the planning of services for each child. As children get older, they may become more directly involved in stating their own opinions and thoughts, providing vital information about their condition and areas of satisfaction or concern with their care coordination. **Objective examination,** an initial and continuing part of any pediatric plan of intervention, is comprised of three basic procedures: screening, evaluation, and assessment. Each of these has a distinct purpose in determining a child's need for intervention (Table 7-2).

Table 7-2: Components of Objective Examination in Pediatric Physical Therapy

Component	Description	Example
Screening	Short, inexpensive tests used to distinguish those children with behaviors that are different from other children of the same age which may indicate the need for further evaluation.	Denver II Developmental Screening Test[31]
Evaluation	Instruments used to gain a comprehensive profile of a child's physical, cognitive, social, emotional, communication, and adaptive abilities to assist in determining therapeutic service needs as well as act as a guide for initial frequency and duration of service.	Bayley II Scales of Infant Development[9]
Assessment	An ongoing process of professional/parent collaboration which begins with the initial screen or evaluation and continues until therapy services are no longer required. Involves the use of both formal and informal mechanisms through which the child's ongoing strengths and needs are determined in a variety of developmental and functional areas.	Pediatric Evaluation of Disability Inventory[38]

Depending on the availability and type of diagnosis at the time of referral, **screening** may or may not be required as an initial objective measurement. Screening is usually indicated when there is risk of a developmental delay or disability. Screening is a quick way to determine if a child is in need of further diagnostic services.

If a child has a definite diagnosis, screening is generally bypassed and a comprehensive evaluation is recommended. **Evaluation** measures are used to gain more in-depth information regarding the child's strengths and needs in all developmental domains. In the case of an orthopaedic condition, this may entail an evaluation of posture or movement as well as special diagnostic tests such as radiographs. Evaluation for the child with a developmental disability is generally obtained through **standardized testing.** This refers to a type of formal test in which the evaluation procedures remain the same when administered by different therapists and at variable test locations. There are a large variety and number of standardized evaluation tests available for pediatric testing, and these are targeted according to the specific purpose of the evaluation (Fig. 7-6).

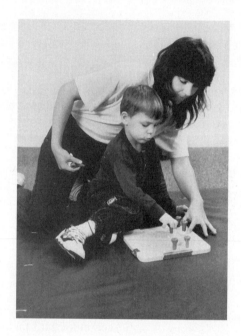

Fig. 7-6. Standardized evaluation: assessment of eye-hand coordination and fine motor skills (Photo credit: Bruce Wang).

In addition to choosing an evaluation which meets the needs of the child being tested, it is also imperative to review each measure for: (1) validity or the ability of the test to measure the content area(s) it claims to measure (e.g., evaluation of mobility); (2) reliability, the consistency of the test between separate administrations or examiners; and (3) the appropriateness of the instrument for the individual disability or culture of the child being assessed (normative group). An equally important element of objective measurement is the information provided through the observations of a child's caregivers in a variety of natural environments (home, daycare, school).

The use of subjective and objective examinations often confirms, revises, or establishes a diagnosis. Determination of a diagnostic condition can be vital information for the child, family, and medical professionals. In many cases, it provides a mechanism by which physical therapists can determine treatment prerogatives and design therapy goals. With certain conditions that have defined physical manifestations, initial therapy can be planned to counteract negative physical outcomes. Diagnosis is also important in order to determine clinical conditions that pose contraindications to specific treatment regimens. There are several positive outcomes associated with establishing a clinical diagnosis, as well as negative outcomes, many of which are based on psychological and social ramifications (Table 7-3). With all children, their families, and friends, the impact of childhood disablement is multi-faceted, and all of those who are touched by it continually experience the many phases of grief and acceptance.

Table 7-3: Outcomes of Establishing a Diagnosis for a Pediatric Patient

Positive Outcomes	Negative Outcomes
• Ability to establish prognosis (future)	• May lead to negative stereotype (label)
• Validates need for services/supports	• May disenfranchise child from obtaining certain services
• May indicate need for genetic counseling	• May cause state of depression or denial
• Assists in possible prevention of disabilities	• False positive diagnosis has negative immediate consequences for both child and family
• Knowledge may assist family with coping mechanisms	• False negative diagnosis will have long term consequences for both child and family
• Aids research efforts targeted for specific conditions	

Prior to the initiation of therapeutic intervention, individualized goals and objectives are developed using the combined information from the family assessment, child observations, and standardized evaluation. The SOAP note format is rarely used as a documentation method for the pediatric patient, with the possible exception of specific hospital or rehabilitation settings (see Chapters 2 and 9 re: SOAP note). Instead, the necessary information is contained in an **Individualized Family Service Plan (IFSP)** or an **Individualized Education Plan (IEP)** developed for each child. These plans are reviewed on a regular basis as the framework for treatment and serve as a baseline by which progress is monitored.

As the name implies, the IFSP describes in detail the total plan of care for the child in the context of the family unit.[26,51] This type of plan, designed for the child from birth to three years of age, is always determined in collaboration with the family where therapeutic needs are intertwined with family needs and priorities. This recognizes that the family unit must remain healthy to provide optimum care for the child. The IFSP might include services such as special baby-sitting assistance, transportation provisions or specialized medical care at home. The IFSP also includes the different therapeutic services that the child will receive, the specific duration and frequency of these services, as well as location of the intervention.

Upon entry into the school system, physical therapy objectives shift to interface with an educational service delivery system and become part of the Individualized Education Plan (IEP). Through this model, therapists often interface with the family, educators, and other health team members to provide direct intervention in the classroom setting.[32,43] The physical therapist (PT) may work individually with the child, in a group setting, or may serve in the role of a consultant to direct care providers. In the latter case, the PT instructs persons who directly care for the child. Instruction may include certain positioning or movement techniques, which will provide therapeutic benefit throughout the day. Regardless of the environment, treatment should be provided in a context in which activities can be targeted to achieve the manner or quality of movement desired.

Young children may be seen by a physical therapist at a variety of locations with different therapist/child ratios, depending on the particular objectives of therapy. Generally, the site of choice is the child's most natural environment which may be the home, school, or a day care setting. Therapists may choose to work with a child in a 1:1 ratio, or in a group with other children, or with the parents. Often some mixture of formats and environments provides treatment variety and the greatest benefit for the child.

It is important to remember that the initiation of therapy does not signal the end of evaluation. Evaluation is an ongoing process which begins with the initial evaluation and continues throughout each therapy session. It includes both subjective and objective examinations of each child's strengths and needs and evolves as the child, family, and therapist continue to determine appropriate therapeutic activities. Annual or bi-annual re-evaluation is extremely important in order to monitor the child's progress and alter therapy goals if necessary. Based on a combination of all assessment information, the health care team and family work in a partnership to determine a well coordinated plan of care for each child.

TREATMENT
PRINCIPLES AND
TECHNIQUES

Treatment in pediatric physical therapy involves assisting each child in gaining abilities which will help him or her meet the daily challenges of the most natural environments. As mentioned earlier, the initial task of the therapist, in collaboration with the family, is an assessment of the child's individual strengths and needs. Using this information, a unique plan and set of goals is developed to facilitate skills in needed areas. Depending on the child's needs or diagnosis, treatment may involve a variety of approaches. The following will detail several methods used to treat children with common orthopaedic and neurological conditions.

In order to initiate therapy with pediatric orthopaedic patients, it is useful to have specific knowledge in the area of pediatric orthopaedics (Box 7-1).[3] Orthopaedic assessment and treatment will vary by condition, but include certain procedures which are common to all orthopaedic clients such as measurement of range of motion (ROM), muscle and sensory testing, gait assessment and postural evaluation. (See Chapter 9, Orthopaedic Physical Therapy, for a further description of these procedures.) Children may require specialized orthopaedic management for acute and long-term orthopaedic conditions as well as neuromuscular diseases. Treatment in both cases requires knowledge of the specific diagnoses as well as protocols for management. For example, specialized surgical procedures often require the therapist to have knowledge of specific post-operative management protocols (e.g., positioning) in order to maintain the surgical correction. Often physical therapists are requested to fabricate splints or casts for the pediatric patient to assist in muscle lengthening or joint stabilization (Fig. 7-7).

Box 7-1

Knowledge Base for Pediatric Orthopaedic Assessment and Treatment*

- Normal pediatric biomechanical alignment
- Specific orthopaedic assessment procedures
- Pre-surgical evaluation of posture and movement
- Post-operative management of specialized surgical interventions
- Rationale and indications/contraindications for using manual therapy
- Use of casts and orthotics for correction or management of musculoskeletal malalignment
- Appropriate use of modalities and exercise protocols for children

*   From Pediatric Orthopaedics, Alexandria, VA, 1992, American Physical Therapy Association.

In addition to orthopaedic techniques, physical therapists use a range of therapeutic techniques which further enhance the rehabilitation process. A variety of neuromotor approaches are used to treat the child with neurological and orthopaedic disabilities. These approaches were primarily developed between 1950 and 1980 and were originally based on the theory, literature, and patient observations during that time frame. These approaches are now being reviewed and adapted in light of current nervous system theories.[54,74] A primary task for both new and veteran pediatric physical therapists is to continue to research the effectiveness of each approach for its use in a variety of settings and in its ability to facilitate the neuromotor changes which they purport. It is also imperative that physical therapists evaluate the effectiveness of each approach in facilitating the child's achievement of targeted goals.

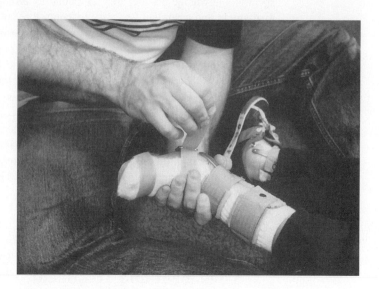

Fig. 7-7. An ankle-foot orthosis is used to assist the orthopaedic needs of a child (Photo credit: Bruce Wang).

Most pediatric physical therapists rely on an "eclectic" or multiple method approach when providing therapy. An **eclectic approach** includes some combination of therapeutic approaches used by the physical therapist and thought to be useful for treatment of a given client.[18] Although the common use of eclectic practice has made it difficult to isolate and study the effectiveness of each specific approach, numerous articles have been published discussing both the controversial nature and effectiveness of a variety of neuromotor approaches.[25,33-35,41-42,58-60] Additional clinical research is necessary in order to achieve a sound basis of support for the continued use of many therapeutic approaches.

At present, a variety of approaches continue to be used in an effort to habilitate and rehabilitate the pediatric client. The following brief descriptions provide an objective overview of the more common neuromotor approaches currently in use.

Neurodevelopmental Treatment Approach (NDT)

This approach was originated by Berta and Karel Bobath in England almost 50 years ago to both analyze and treat neurological disorders of posture and movement.[13,15,16] Through the use of a motivating environment and a child's active participation, manual facilitation and inhibition techniques are employed by the therapist to present the child with a "normal" sensory experience thereby encouraging facilitation of a more functional motor response.[11,14,15] Continued active repetition of normal developmental skills assists the child in establishing more coordinated, efficient movement patterns.[11,14,16] Implemented throughout the world by therapists, parents, teachers and other professionals, NDT is the most widely used and documented therapeutic approach in the United States for the treatment of upper motor neuron lesions, such as cerebral palsy (Fig. 7-8).[23,29]

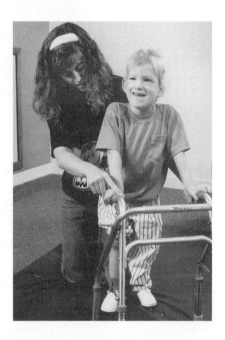

Fig. 7-8. A child ambulates with facilitation from the therapist (Photo credit: Bruce Wang).

Sensory Integration Theory (SI)

This technique is based on the theory that poor integration and use of sensory input (feedback) prevents subsequent motor planning (output). The SI approach assesses the child's sensory systems through clinical observations and tests prior to initiation of therapy. Providing controlled vestibular and somatosensory experiences enables the child to integrate the sensory information to evoke a spontaneous, functional response (Fig. 7-9).[4,58]

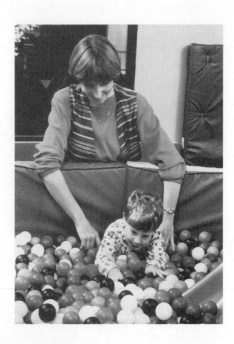

Fig. 7-9. Sensory integration can be fun (Photo credit: Bruce Wang).

Normal Developmental Theory

Therapy goals and objectives are designed to follow the progression of normal motor development (developmental milestones) as well as developmental theory (e.g., development proceeds proximal to distal). The approach is based on a model of higher level cortical control which dictates the maturation process. The theory assumes that children with central nervous system damage will acquire motor skills in a similar fashion as children with normally developing nervous systems.[18] Many of the neuromotor therapies used today were originally based on this theoretical foundation.[19]

Conductive Education

Founded by Andras Pèto in Budapest, Hungary, almost 40 years ago, this approach is based on the original motor learning concepts of Bernstein and Luria as well as the works of Piaget in which disability is a result of the interaction between the child and the environment.[12,39] One individual (a conductor) works with the child as an active learner by assisting her or him with completion of all daily activities while the child repeats rhythmic, verbal phrases describing her/his actions.[40] Implemented primarily outside of the United States, this approach is used to promote maximal independence while accomplishing daily functional tasks within the child's scope of abilities.[62]

CASE STUDIES: THE MANY FACES OF PEDIATRIC PHYSICAL THERAPY

Matthew

Matthew is three years old and is one of many preschoolers at the Rosedale Preschool. Matthew has Downs syndrome.

Matthew attends preschool with other infants and toddlers. He plays with balls and puzzles and loves to swim. Administration of a formal evaluation revealed Matthew has many strengths as well as needs in the gross and fine motor domains. Matthew is severely hypotonic (low muscle tone) and has difficulty running without falling. This was noted on the formal evaluation as well as in observations by Matthew's parents and preschool teacher. It was also noted that his automatic reactions to disturbances of balance (righting reactions and protective responses) were delayed, especially when moving in and out of various positions (transitions). Matthew was able to grasp objects in a manner appropriate for other three-year-olds and enjoys drawing and playing with building blocks. He continues to exhibit needs in feeding skills due to the low muscle tone in the muscles used for chewing and mouth closure. His medical history reveals Matthew has a congenital heart problem as well as several other distinguishing features associated with Downs syndrome.

Research has attempted to determine appropriate physical therapy intervention for the child with Downs syndrome.[70] Drawing conclusions from this research, it appears most important to provide a child with Downs syndrome opportunities to explore a variety of environments requiring different postural adjustments or movement patterns. In accordance with this, the therapist must observe the individual motor learning style of each child, and respond to this by creating challenging learning situations.

In Matthew's case, the physical therapist will provide therapy in the school as designed in his Individualized Education Plan, and collaborate with his preschool staff by instructing them to carry out physical therapy goals throughout his daily school routine. An inclusion program such as the one at Rosedale Preschool, maintains a philosophy that children with a variety of developmental abilities should play and learn together in an atmosphere which fosters a sense of belonging and personal growth for all its members. This is naturally where a child who is as special as Matthew belongs.

Matthew's Individualized Education Plan. Due to Matthew's diagnosis of congenital heart disease, it is important that he avoid excessive exertion and fatigue. Activities that involve impact to the cervical vertebrae should also be avoided due to his vertebral instability. In designing a plan for Matthew, consideration is placed primarily on family goals and Matthew's current interests. It is from this frame of reference that therapeutic goals and objectives will be designed. Specific objectives might involve achieving a task that is appropriate for Matthew's developmental abilities as well as his functional level. Most objectives target a particular skill, the manner of performance or assistance, and criterion to be met (Box 7-2).

Box 7-2

Example of a Goal and Criterion for Matthew

Goal: Matthew will run across a level (hard) mat surface without falling when prompted with his favorite toy.

Criterion: Three to four times during four play sessions.

The same skill can also be scaled[61] so that Matthew will always achieve different measures of success and his individual progress can be followed over time (Box 7-3). Initial therapeutic goals are vital in order to assess treatment response as well as to maintain treatment consistency. Through the ongoing assessment process, Matthew's progress will be monitored with alterations made to his care plan if warranted.

Box 7-3

Goal Attainment Scaling

-2   Matthew will walk across the level mat surface without falling when prompted with his favorite toy.

-1   Matthew will run across the level mat surface with one stop to regain his balance (hands down on mat) when prompted with his favorite toy.

 0   Matthew will run across the level mat surface without falling when prompted with his favorite toy.

+1   Matthew will run across a mat angled 10 degrees with one stop to regain his balance (hands down on mat) when prompted with his favorite toy.

+2   Matthew will run across a mat raised by a 10-degree angle without a stop or fall when prompted with his favorite toy.

Intervention. Physical therapy intervention may first involve assisting Matthew in developing a relationship with his environment. Matthew may initially move too quickly or slowly, take steps which are too large or uneven or resist the challenge to ambulate altogether. During the activity, the therapist may use NDT techniques such as guided handling to assist with movement. Another strategy may involve Matthew's active participation through the use of cognitive and verbal reinforcement during the motor activity to reinforce learning.

As mentioned previously, some combination of techniques may best accomplish the task (See Treatment Principles and Techniques). If each of Matthew's goals can be designed according to his motivations (e.g., eating, play), the inclusion of therapeutic approaches and techniques becomes more functional and likely to meet with success.

Emmie

Emmie began her life in the Neonatal Intensive Care Unit (NICU) of Eastern Shore Memorial Hospital. Her first experiences were the sounds of the slow beeps and hums of the infant monitors. Her first visions were obstructed by glass and her human touch limited to those persons performing routine checks of her medical status. Unlike other newborn infants who experience the sounds of home and arms of friends or siblings, Emmie will have to wait until she has surgery because she was born with "spina bifida" (Meningomyelocele—see Common Conditions). Children with spina bifida and their families have no choice but to begin their lives in the hospital environment. Despite diligent efforts, which have improved the comfort and familiarity of hospital NICUs and pediatric units, they continue to be a threatening, imposing environment for families.

Management. The general goals of physical therapy management for Emmie and other children with spina bifida are: (1) to prevent physiological impairment from becoming a disability, which is the functional consequence of an impairment (e.g., "can't crawl"); and (2) to improve the quality of life for each child and family by preventing a disability from becoming a handicap, which is the social consequence of a disability (e.g., "can't go to the school dance").[44] Accomplishing these goals requires a collaborative approach between the child, the family, and the health care team. Physical therapy assessment should be comprehensive and interface closely with the observations and assessments of other health care team and family members. Assessment and continued follow-up (monitoring) should include the following specific objectives:

- General multidomain screen and evaluation of developmental level
- Neurological evaluation, including monitoring for signs of increased intracranial pressure
- Orthopaedic assessment for joint range and mobility, kyphosis, scoliosis or dislocations
- Assessment of bowel and bladder function
- Assessment of skin integrity
- Activities of Daily Living (ADL)
- Assessment of mobility

Emmie's Individualized Family Service Plan. Activities are generally centered around the goals and objectives indicated in each child's individualized plan. For a child Emmie's age, the format would likely be an Individualized Family Service Plan (IFSP). The child with spina bifida often presents with a range of cognitive delays and skills in the psychosocial area. Consideration of these abilities, as well as physical and environmental factors, are all essential when designing a plan of care. During the first few years of life, Emmie will develop a sense of her autonomy and self esteem, therefore physical therapy will focus on her ability to explore her environment.

Depending on each child's abilities, the physical therapist will explore options to accomplish mobility goals. Many children with spina bifida use orthotics or braces to assist in locomotion. A popular choice for the young child is the parapodium. This upright brace positions the child in standing on a flat swivel base with unencumbered arms and hands, allowing the child freedom to explore the environment.[50] Therapy goals may also focus on position transitions, muscle strengthening, and self-care activities. As Emmie reaches adolescence, she will likely choose to use a wheelchair, which allows greater speed and efficiency for daily living. She may continue to be seen on a periodic basis through the hospital's outpatient clinic or opt for private outpatient care. Therapy will continue only on an "as needed" basis to assist with problems which arise during transitional developmental phases.

SUMMARY

Physical therapists who work with pediatric patients focus on child development, psychology, and learning. They may provide services to the patient for a long period of time, a short period, or on a consultant basis. Intervention is family centered and usually incorporates activities adapted to play. Physical therapy is frequently rendered in the school setting as directed by federal entitlement programs.

Common conditions seen by pediatric physical therapists are generally classified as orthopaedic, genetic, chromosomal, or environmentally related disorders. Screening, evaluation, and assessment techniques are employed to establish goals and objectives which are incorporated into an Individualized Family Services Plan or Individualized Education Plan. Treatment is often eclectic, that is, it combines components from a variety of approaches including neurodevelopmental treatment, sensory integration, normal developmental theory, and motor learning theory (conductive education).

Pediatric physical therapy is challenging and rewarding. Research, legislation, and new techniques create a changing practice environment to enhance the quality of care. The result is an exciting specialty in physical therapy.

References

1. Allen MC and Capute AJ: Neonatal neurodevelopmental examination as a predictor of neuromotor outcome in premature infants, Pediatrics 83(4):498-506, 1989.

2. American Academy of Pediatrics: Committee on Sports Medicine: atlantoaxial instability in Downs syndrome, Pediatrics 74(1):152-154, 1984.

3. Pediatric Orthopedics, Alexandria, VA, 1992, American Physical Therapy Association.

4. Ayres AJ: Sensory integration and learning disorders, Los Angeles, CA, 1972, Western Psychological Services.

5. Bailey D, Simeonsson R, editors: Family assessment in early intervention: Rationale and model for family assessment in early intervention, Columbus, OH, 1988 Merrill Publishing Company.

6. Barden HS: Growth and development of selected hard tissues in Downs syndrome: a review, Hum Biol 55:539-576, 1983.

7. Batshaw M, Perret Y, Shapiro B: Normal and abnormal development. In Batshaw M, Perret Y: Children with disabilities: a medical primer, ed 3 Baltimore, 1992, Brookes Publishing Company.

8. Batshaw M, Perret Y: Bones, joints, and muscles: support and movement. In Batshaw M, Perret Y: Children with disabilities: a medical primer, Baltimore, 1992, Brookes Publishing Company.

9. Bayley N: Bayley scales of infant development, New York, 1969, The Psychological Corporation.

10. Blackman JA: Medical aspects of developmental disabilities in children birth to three, ed 2, Rockville, 1990, Aspen Publishers.

11. Bly A: Historical and current view of the basis of NDT, Ped Phys Ther 3(3):131-135, 1991.

12. Bernstein N: The coordination and regulation of movements, Oxford, UK, 1967, Pergamon Press.

13. Bobath, B: A neurodevelopmental treatment of cerebral palsy, Physiotherapy 49:242-244, 1963.

14. Bobath K, Bobath B: Facilitation of normal postural reactions and movement in the treatment of cerebral palsy. Physiotherapy. 50:246-262, 1964.

15. Bobath B, Bobath K: The neuro-developmental treatment. In Sutton D, editor: Management of motor disorders in children with cerebral palsy, Philadelphia, 1984, JB Lippincott Company.

16. Bobath K: A neurophysiological basis for the treatment of cerebral palsy, Philadelphia, 1980, JB Lippincott Company.

17. Bottos M, et al: Locomotor strategies preceding independent walking: prospective study of neurological and language development in 424 cases. Dev Med Child Neurol 31(1):25-34, 1989.

18. Campbell PH: Posture and movement. In Tingey C editor: Implementing early intervention, Baltimore, MD, 1989, Paul H Brookes.

19. Campbell PH, Finn D: Programming to influence acquisition of motor abilities in infants and young children, Ped Phys Ther 3:200-205, 1991.

20. Cassidy JT, Petty RE: Textbook of pediatric rheumatology, ed 2, New York, 1990, Churchill Livingston.

21. Chasnoff IJ, Burns KA, & Burns WJ: Cocaine use in pregnancy: perinatal morbidity and mortality, Neurotoxicol Teratol 9(4):291-293, 1987.

22. Cherry DB: Pediatric physical therapy: philosophy, science and techniques, Ped Phys Ther (3)2:70-76, Summer, 1991.

23. Conner F, Williamson G, Sieff JA: Programming for the infants and toddlers with neuromotor and other developmental disabilities, New York, 1978, Teachers College Press.

24. Cooley WC, Graham JM, Jr: Common syndromes and management issues for primary care physicians: Downs syndrome: an update and review for the primary pediatrician, Clin Pediatr 30(4):233-253, 1991.

25. Cotton E: Improvement of motor function with the use of conductive education, Dev Med Child Neurol 16(5):637-643, 1974.

26. Deal A, Dunst C: A flexible and functional approach to developing individualized family support plans. Infants and Young Children 1(4):32-43, 1989.

27. Doberczak TM, et al: Neonatal neurologic and electroencephalographic effects of intrauterine cocaine exposure, J Pediatr 113(2):354-358, 1988.

28. Education of All Handicapped Children Act of 1975, Public Law 94-142, 20 U. S. C. 1401, 1975.

29. Finnie N: Handling your young cerebral palsied child at home. New York, 1975, Dutton.

30. Foster M, Phillips W: Family systems theory as a framework for problem solving in pediatric physical therapy, Ped Phys Ther 4:70-73, 1992.

31. Frankenburg WK: Denver developmental screening test manual, Denver CO, 1973, LADOCA Project & Publishing Foundation.

32. Giangreco M: Delivery of therapeutic services in special education programs for learners with severe handicaps, Phys Occupa Ther Pediatr 6:5-15, 1986.

33. Golden GS: Nonstandard therapies in the developmental disabilities, American Journal of Diseases of Children 134(5):487-491, 1980.

34. Golden GS: Controversial therapies in developmental disabilities. In Gottlieb MI, Williams JE, editors: Developmental-Behavioral Disorders: Selected Topics (Vol. 3). New York, 1990, Plenum.

35. Goodgold-Edwards SA: Principles for guiding action during motor learning: A critical evaluation of neurodevelopmental treatment, Phys Ther Prac 2(4):30-39, 1993.

36. Graham JM: Independent dysmorphology evaluations at birth and 4 years of age for children exposed to varying amounts of alcohol in utero. Pediatrics, 81(6):772-778, 1988.

37. Guccione A: Physical therapy diagnosis and the relationship between impairments and function, Phys Ther 71(7):499-503, 1991.

38. Haley SM, et al: Pediatric evaluation of disability inventory (PEDI): development, standardization and administration manual, Boston, 1992, New England Medical Center Hospitals and PEDI Research Group.

39. Hari M: The human principle in conductive education. Budapest, Hungary, 1988, International Peto Institute.

40. Hari M, Tillemans T: Conductive education (Clinics in Developmental Medicine No. 90). In Scrutton D, editor: Management of the motor disorders of children with cerebral palsy, Oxford, England, 1984, Blackwell Scientific Publications.

41. Harris S: Early intervention: does developmental therapy make a difference? Topics Early Childhood Special Education 7:20-32, 1988.

42. Harris SR, et al: Accepted and controversial neuromotor therapies for infants at high risk for cerebral palsy, J Perinatol 8(1):3-13, 1987.

43. Henry B: The role of physical therapists in development of individualized educational plans, Totline 12: 13-15, 1986.

44. Hirst M: Patterns of impairment and disability related to social handicap in young people with cerebral palsy and spina bifida, J Biosoc Sci 21:1-12, 1989.

45. Hyser CL, Mendell JR: Recent advances in Duchenne and Becker muscular dystrophy. Neurol Clin 6(3):429-453, 1988.

46. Individuals with Disabilities Education Act Amendments of 1991, Public Law 102-119, 105 STAT.587, 1991.

47. International classification of impairment, disability and handicap, Geneva, Switzerland, 1980, World Health Organization.

48. Lawrence KM: Neural tube defects: a two-pronged approach to primary prevention, Pediatrics 70(4):648-650, 1982.

49. Linder TW: Transdiciplinary play-based assessment: a functional approach to working with young children, Baltimore, 1990, Brookes Publishing.

50. Liptak G: Spina bifida in primary pediatric care, Hoekelman, RA, editor: St. Louis, 1992, Mosby-Yearbook Inc.

51. McGonigel M, Garland C: The individualized family service plan and the early intervention team: team and family issues and recommended practices. Infants and Young Children 1(1):10-21, 1988.

52. Mills JL, Graubard BI: Is moderate drinking during pregnancy associated with an increased risk of malformations? Pediatrics 80(3):309-314, 1987.

53. Mills JL: The absence of a relation between the pericon-ceptional use of vitamins and neural-tube defects. N Eng J Med 321(7):430-435, 1989.

54. Montgomery P: Neurodevelopmental treatment and sensory integrative theory. In Lister MJ, editor: Contemporary management and motor control problems: Proceedings from the II Step conference, Alexandria, VA, 1991, Foundation for Physical Therapy.

55. MRC Vitamin Study Research Group: Prevention of neural tube defects: results of the medical research council vitamin study, Lancet 338(8760):131-137, 1991.

56. National Maternal & Child Health Resource Center: Community-based service systems for children with special health care needs and their families, US Surgeon General's Conference Campaign '88, September, 1988.

57. Newald J: Cocaine infants: A new arrival at hospital's step? Hospitals 60(7):96, 1986.

58. Ottenbacher K: Sensory integration therapy: affect or effect. Am J Occup Ther 36(9):571-578, 1982.

59. Ottenbacher KJ, et al: Quantitative analysis of the effectiveness of pediatric therapy: emphasis on neurodevelopmental treatment approach. Phys Ther 66:1095-1101, 1986.

60. Palisano R: Research on the effectiveness of neurodevelopmental treatment, Ped Phys Ther 3(3):143-148, 1991.

61. Palisano R, et al: Goal attainment scaling as a measure of change in infants with motor delays, Phys Ther 72(6):432-437, 1992.

62. Pueschel SM: Clinical aspects of Downs syndrome from infancy to adulthood, Am J Med Genet 7(suppl.):52-56, 1990.

63. Roche AF: The cranium in Mongolism, Acta Neurologica 42:62-78, 1966.

64. Rommens JM, et al: Identification of the cystic fibrosis gene: chromosome walking and jumping, Science 245(4922):1059-1065, 1989.

65. Scher MS, et al: Destructive brain lesions of presumed fetal onset: Antepartum causes of cerebral palsy, Pediatrics 88(5):898-906, 1991.

66. Schneider JW: Motor assessment and parent education beyond the newborn period. In Chasnoff IJ editor: Drugs, alcohol, pregnancy and parenting, Lancaster, UK, 1988, Kluwer.

67. Schneider JW, Chasnoff IJ: Cocaine abuse during pregnancy: its effects on infant motor development - a clinical perspective, Topics in Acute Care and Trauma Rehabilitation 2:59-69, 1987.

68. Schneider JW, Griffith DR, Chasnoff IJ: Infants exposed to cocaine in utero: implications for developmental assessment and intervention, Infants and Young Children 2(1):25-36, 1989.

69. Scull S: Juvenile rheumatoid arthritis. In Tecklin JS, editor: Pediatric physical therapy, Philadelphia, 1994, JB Lippincott Company.

70. Shea AM: Motor attainments in Downs syndrome. In Lister MJ, editor: Contemporary management of motor control problems: Proceedings of the II Step conference, Alexandria, VA, 1991, Foundation for Physical Therapy.

71. Spicer RL: Cardiovascular disease in Downs syndrome. Pediatr Clin North Am 31(6):1331-1343, 1984.

72. Streissguth AP, et al: Attention, distraction and reaction time at age 7 years and prenatal alcohol exposure, Neurobehav Toxicol and Teratol 8(6):717-725, 1986.

73. Styer-Acevedo J: Physical therapy for the child with cerebral palsy. In Tecklin JS, editor, Pediatric physical therapy, Philadelphia, 1994, JB Lippincott Company.

74. Umphred D: Merging neurophysiologic approaches with contemporary theories. In Lister MJ, editor: Contemporary management of motor control problems: Proceedings from the II Step conference, Alexandria, VA, 1991, Foundation for Physical Therapy.

75. U.S. Department of Health and Human Services: Public Health Service, Surgeon General's Report, Children with Special Health Care Needs, Campaign '87 11, June, 1987.

76. Wessel HB: Spinal muscular atrophy, Pediatric Ann 18(7):421-427, 1989.

Review Questions

1. Distinguish the three levels of the WHO continuum of disablement. Create scenarios to demonstrate examples of each level.

2. For the brief, comprehensive purposes of this chapter, suggest broad practice approaches that would probably be in violation of Public Law 99-457 (e.g., activities which would not support family centered and environmental aspects of treatment).

3. Describe what is meant by a developmental delay. Identify fetal risk factors.

4. Define juvenile rheumatoid arthritis and describe how distinct subtypes might vary. Speculate on how these variations might affect treatment approach, creating a brief scenario to illustrate your point.

5. Create a list of assessment process strategies or procedures and identify them as either *screening, evaluation,* or *assessment* tools.

6. Describe the kinds of questions you might raise in determining whether a selected evaluation measure would be the best one for a given client.

7. Weigh the positive and negative outcomes of a clinical diagnosis, applying them to a specific example.

8. Within the limited scope of this text's purpose, create a situation in which a physical therapist uses an "eclectic approach." Incorporate several of the therapeutic approaches discussed in this chapter.

Chapter 8

Neurological Physical Therapy

Shree Pandya

> " **A** sense of history and an appreciation of why things happened can provide a perspective in understanding the present and in projecting the future. "
>
> Lucy Blair, PT

KEY TERMS

akinesia
amyotrophic lateral sclerosis (ALS)
angiography
bradykinesia
Brunnstrom's approach
computerized axial tomography (CAT or CT scan)
electroencephalography (EEG)
electromyography (EMG)
expressive aphasia
hypertonia
hypotonia
lumbar puncture
magnetic resonance imaging (MRI)
motor control

motor learning
multiple sclerosis (MS)
nerve conduction velocity (NCV) studies
paraplegia
Parkinson's disease
perception
proprioceptive neuromuscular facilitation (PNF)
quadraplegia
receptive aphasia
rigidity
Rood's approach
sensation
spinal cord injuries (SCI)
stroke or cerebrovascular accident (CVA)
tone
traumatic brain injury (TBI)
tremor

GENERAL DESCRIPTION

The 1990s were declared the decade of the brain by the United States Congress. In fact, since the 1980s, tremendous progress has been made in the areas of neuroscience, clinical neurology, and genetics. At the beginning of the century, one could learn about the human nervous system from autopsy tissue samples only. Today, with new technologies available, the brain can be seen in action in living human beings. As the function of the brain and nervous system is better understood, so is the field of neurological physical therapy. Physical therapists are better able to understand and explain the effect of each technique used.

Patients with problems related to disorders of the nervous system make up a large proportion of individuals treated by physical therapists today. Disorders of the nervous system can be inherited or acquired. Acquired disorders may result from trauma, disease, secondary to disorders affecting other body systems, or as part of the normal aging process. There are also many disorders affecting the nervous system whose causes are still unknown or not well understood.

Neurologic disorders can affect people at any age. For example, inherited disorders are present from birth. Traumatic disorders like spinal cord injuries or brain injuries are most often caused by motor vehicle accidents, and the age groups most commonly involved range from the teens to the thirties. Disorders like multiple sclerosis, Parkinson's disease, and the muscular dystrophies manifest most often between the thirties to sixties. The two most common neurologic disorders encountered with age are stroke (paralysis secondary to disruption of the blood flow within the brain) and Alzheimer's disease. Thus, when working with patients with neurologic problems, therapists are likely to encounter persons of any age, both sexes, and all races.

Depending on the cause of the disorder, the condition may be lifelong or temporary. It may be reversible, static or progressive. The patient may go through periods of "plateaus" (i.e., relative stability interspersed with progression). Because of the lengthy course of most neurologic disorders, physical therapists have extended contact with their patients and play a critical role in their care. Based on the condition, the stage of illness, and the reason for referral, the frequency of treatment will vary. For example, patients may be treated as often as two times per day for an hour each in the rehabilitation or hospital setting or two to three times per week if the patient is past the acute stage and is being seen in the home or extended care facility. If the therapist sees the patient on a consultation basis or for education regarding personal care and management, these visits may be as infrequently as monthly, quarterly, or on a yearly basis.

From the above description of neurologic practice, it is apparent that physical therapists will no doubt encounter diversity in their patients, work settings, and patient management. This is a major change from the early days of physical therapy practice and even from 20 years ago, when physical therapists practiced under physician orders only and followed prescriptions for massage, electrotherapy, thermal agents, hydrotherapy, and exercises. Today the physical therapist is an autonomous member of the health care team and in many states practices under direct access. The role of the therapist today is to evaluate, treat, and prevent problems, as well as to consult with and educate health care team members, families, and patients regarding those problems. This chapter describes the practice of physical therapy as it relates to disorders of the nervous system.

COMMON CONDITIONS

Stroke

Stroke or **cerebrovascular accident (CVA)** refers to the neurological problems arising from disruption of blood flow in the brain. This disruption may be caused by hemorrhage (bleeding) or a blockage that results in ischaemia (decreased oxygen) due to a clot. The type and severity of symptoms will depend on the area of brain tissue involved. The most common symptom is a complete paralysis or partial weakness on the side opposite the site involved. Depending on the site of the lesion, the paralysis may be accompanied by symptoms such as neglect of the affected side and difficulty speaking or understanding the spoken word. Approximately 30 percent of patients die during the first month. Of the survivors, approximately 30 to 40 percent will have severe disability.[9] A major psychological problem post-stroke is depression, which can have a great impact on management. Recovery from stroke occurs most rapidly during the first six months, but functional gains can be seen for up to two years or longer.

The purpose of physical therapy is to facilitate and enhance functional recovery occurring in response to the resolution of neurologic changes. Once functional recovery plateaus, the therapist and assistant will teach the patient and family to adapt and compensate for the residual deficits in order to function at the optimal level possible within the constraints of the condition.

Figures 8-1 and 8-2 illustrate the preventive and functional training aspects of management respectively for a patient with left-sided paralysis due to a stroke.

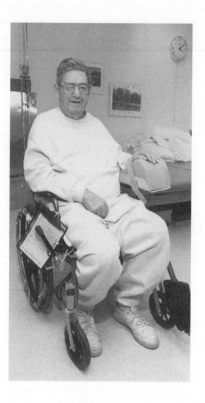

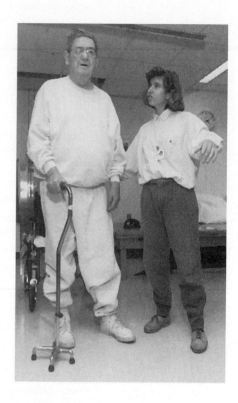

Fig. 8-1. Positioning for a patient with a stroke to prevent secondary problems in shoulder and hand on the paralyzed (left) side.

Fig. 8-2. Gait training for a patient with left-sided paralysis due to a stroke.

Traumatic Brain Injury

Traumatic brain injury (TBI) is most often caused during motor vehicle accidents or due to falls and violence.[7] Because of the nature of the injury, there may be fractures, dislocations, lacerations, etc., associated with brain trauma. The groups most commonly affected are children and young adults, with TBI being the most common cause of death and disability in this age group. Early management is focused on preservation of life and prevention of further damage. The diffuse nature of the brain injury usually results in problems with multiple brain functions and mechanisms. A complex picture is common, with varying deficits in motor and sensory capabilities, intellectual and cognitive functions, and emotional and psychological functions. Because of the complexity and variability of problems that may be encountered with each patient, management and treatment require an individualized plan and a multidisciplinary team approach in which each team member plays a specific and significant role. Currently, there is not enough data available about long-term outcomes or valid and reliable measures that may help predict outcomes. Hence, this area provides several opportunities for research to answer questions important to patients and their families.

Spinal Cord Injury

Spinal cord injuries (SCI), like traumatic brain injuries, most often result from motor vehicle accidents, falls, violence (especially gun shot wounds), and sports (diving and football). The age group most often affected is between 15–25 years of age and men are affected four times as much as women.[12] Spinal cord damage can occur due to other diseases and conditions also, and in those instances, older patients are affected more commonly. Depending on the level of injury, all limbs may be affected **(quadriplegia)** or the lower trunk and legs may be affected **(paraplegia).** If the lesion is complete, there is no residual sensory or motor function below the level of the lesion (-plegia). When the cord is not completely severed, some distal motor and/or sensory functions may be preserved (-paresis).

As with TBI, SCI may be accompanied by multiple injuries and the early goal of management is preservation of life and prevention of further damage to the neural tissue. Further damage is prevented through internal immobilization of the area by fusing the vertebrae with bone grafts, rods, and wires—or externally with devices like body jackets or casts.

While this healing process occurs, it is important to maintain mobility in the joints of the extremities, strength in the unaffected muscles, cardiorespiratory capacity, and endurance. Figure 8-3 illustrates one of the types of body jackets used to provide stability. The patient is working on strengthening the upper extremity and trunk muscles. Once medical and orthopaedic clearance is obtained, more vigorous functional training is begun.

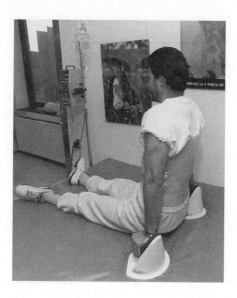

Fig. 8-3. Patient with spinal cord injury in a body jacket, working on upper body strengthening.

As illustrated in Figures 8-4 and 8-5, the patients are learning mat table-to-wheelchair transfers and wheelchair manipulation skills. Simultaneously, equipment needs and environmental adaptations need to be identified. For example, most patients use a wheelchair as a primary means of mobility. These need to be custom ordered for each patient with specific size and adaptation requirements. Figure 8-6 shows a patient with quadriplegia using an electric wheelchair for mobility and a special device that allows him to write. The home will need to be made accessible to the chair with ramps and other modifications. Thus, a therapist plays a major role not only in the treatment, but also management, of patients with SCI by providing family education and consultation on many related issues.

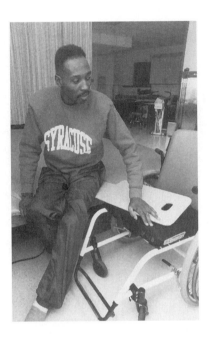

Fig. 8-4. Patient with paraplegia working on mat table-to-wheelchair transfers.

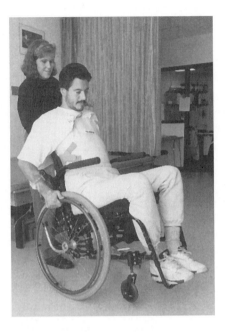

Fig. 8-5. Patient with paraplegia working on wheelchair manipulation skills necessary for going up and down curbs.

Multiple Sclerosis

Multiple sclerosis (MS) is a disease in which patches of demyelination occur in the nervous system, leading to disturbances in conduction of messages along the nerves. The condition most often manifests between the ages of 15 and 45 years, affecting women more often than men. The specific cause is still unknown. The disease can present with a variety of symptoms based on the location of the patches of nerve demyelination. Common symptoms include weakness, fatigue, alteration in sensation, disturbances of eye movements, and speech. The course in the early stages is unpredictable. Eventually, the course may take one of four forms:[8] (1) benign, in which the disease seems to go into remission, and the patient is relatively symptom-free, with no functional disabilities; (2) exacerbating-remitting, in which the patient undergoes periods of worsening followed by periods of improvement; (3) remitting-progressive, which is similar to the above except that improvement after the worsening is not as complete and each episode leaves a residual problem or increase in problems, causing a general progression of the disease; and (4) progressive, in which the disease progresses unremittingly, causing severe disability.

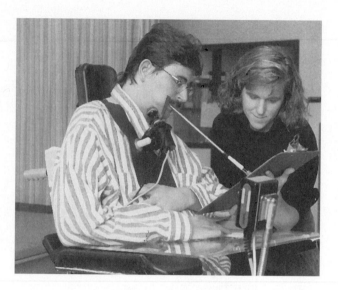

Fig. 8-6. Patient with quadriplegia in a customized electric chair using a special device that enables him to write.

The role of the therapist with this group of patients is more consultative and educational. Patients may benefit from active treatment during an acute exacerbation but otherwise require periodic evaluations and recommendations based on their changing functional needs.

Parkinson's Disease

This is a progressive condition first described by James Parkinson in 1817. It is also referred to as paralysis agitans and idiopathic (cause unknown) parkinsonism and is commonly seen with advancing age. **Parkinson's disease** is characterized by a classic triad of symptoms. **Tremor** (alternating contractions of opposing muscle groups), usually affecting the hands and feet, tends to occur at rest (e.g., when the part is not being used or moved). **Rigidity,** a disturbance of muscle tone, manifests as a resistance when the limbs are passively moved. **Bradykinesia,** a slowness of movements, and/or **akinesia,** a poverty of movements, completes the triad.[2]

This condition results from a deficiency of dopamine, a neurotransmitter (chemical messenger) which is produced in a region of the brain called the substantia nigra. The specific cause for this depletion is unknown. Even though a cure is not available, medications that restore the neurochemical balance are available and help alleviate the symptoms. Unfortunately, the effectiveness of the medications diminishes over the years, and the symptoms continue to worsen.

The tremor, rigidity, and bradykinesia have a great impact on the patient's ability to maintain balance and perform activities like walking, stair climbing, reaching, etc. Patients tend to develop a stooped posture, walk with short, shuffling steps, and loose reciprocal arm movements. The role of the therapist is to educate the patient and family about the secondary problems that result from the basic deficits and teach the patient compensatory strategies to maintain function and prevent/minimize further problems.

Amyotrophic Lateral Sclerosis

Amyotrophic lateral sclerosis (ALS), also known as "Lou Gehrig's disease" (after the famous baseball player), is a rapidly progressive neurological disorder associated with a degeneration of the motor nerve cells. Its cause is unknown. The median age of onset is in the fifties.[4] It is characterized by weakness, atrophy (loss of muscle bulk), and fasciculations (muscle twitches). The weakness can be present in the limb muscles (leading to difficulty with functional activities) or in muscles involved with speech, swallowing, and breathing (causing difficulties with those activities). Regardless of where it begins, eventually all muscles are involved. Currently there is no cure for this disease, and the rate of survival is about four years from diagnosis to death.

The role of the therapist is to provide preventive and supportive care for the secondary problems of weakness, to recommend appropriate devices and equipment to keep the patient as independent as possible, and to educate the family and caregivers regarding handling of the patient. (See also Chapter 8, "Pediatric Physical Therapy," and Chapter 11, "Physical Therapy for the Older Adult" for additional neurological conditions common to those age groups.)

EVALUATION PRINCIPLES AND TECHNIQUES

The goal of physical therapy is to improve and/or maintain functional movements and prevent decline. Functional movements include not only the activities of daily living (dressing, eating, bathing, etc.), but also those necessary for educational, vocational, and recreational purposes. Thus, likely candidates for physical therapy are individuals with disorders of movement or function resulting from involvement of the nervous system.

In order to assess the cause of movement dysfunction, the contributing factors need to be examined individually and collectively. Most patients with neurological problems are referred to physical therapy after extensive evaluation by a neurologist and/or physiatrist. The first step in patient evaluation is to review all the pertinent medical records and data. The therapist will need to make note of not only the current conditions and problems, but also any previous problems or current comorbid conditions that will affect the prognosis. The therapist will also need to note psychological, emotional, and social factors that may have an impact.

A therapist needs to be familiar with and understand the results and implications of special tests used by physicians in order to arrive at a diagnosis. Some of the tests commonly used include radiographs (use of x-rays on photographic film), **computerized axial tomography (CAT** or **CT scan**—computer synthesis of x-rays transmitted through a specific plane of the body), **magnetic resonance imaging (MRI**—computer images produced by placing the body part in a magnetic field), angiography, lumbar puncture, and electrodiagnostic tests.[1] The CAT scans and MRIs have only become available during the past two decades as a result of improved (CAT) and new (MRI) technologies. They have revolutionized the diagnostic capabilities by providing three-dimensional and cross-sectional images of internal structures, including the brain and spinal cord. These tests provide better visualization of and differentiation among tissues like bone, nerve cells, and blood as they relate to the brain and spinal cord. **Angiography** involves injecting radiopaque material into the blood vessels to better visualize and identify problems such as occlusion (blockage) of blood vessels, aneurysms, and vascular malformations.

Lumbar puncture is a procedure used for three main purposes: (1) to measure intracranial pressure, (2) to inject a radiopaque substance for a myelograph, or (3) to obtain a sample of the cerebrospinal fluid (CSF) for examination. The procedure is performed under local anesthesia. A needle is inserted in the space between the L_3 and L_4 vertebrae until it reaches the subarachnoid space and then, based on the purpose of the lumbar puncture, the appropriate procedure is performed. The CSF is examined for chemical and cellular content—that is, the specific type and number of cells present. It is also used to identify or obtain bacteriologic or viral cultures.

Electrodiagnostic tests are also very helpful in identifying the neurological disorder. **Electroencephalography (EEG)** involves recording of the electrical potential/activity in the brain by placing electrodes on the scalp. This test is essential in the diagnosis and management of patients with seizure disorders. **Electromyography (EMG)** involves recording the electrical activity in the muscle during a state of rest and during voluntary contraction. It helps differentiate disorders primarily related to muscle pathology and/or secondary to nerve or neuromuscular junction disorders. **Nerve conduction velocity (NCV) studies** involve recording the rate at which electrical signals are transmitted along peripheral nerves. These studies help clarify and differentiate disorders that affect the axons versus those that affect the myelin sheath covering the axons. In many cases, the physical therapist performs the diagnostic tests, such as an EMG or NCV, and provides information directly to the individual.

Knowledge of these tests and the results not only gives the therapist a better understanding of the disorder and its implications and progression, but also enables the therapist to respond appropriately to questions the patient may have about these procedures.

The next step in the evaluation is an interview with the patient or a family member/caregiver. The interview gives the therapist an opportunity to hear first-hand the sequence of events that brought the patient to therapy. It allows the therapist to ask specific questions that will provide information about the patient's pre-morbid (pre-disease) lifestyle and functional level, as well as assess the patient's cognitive and communicative capabilities. The interview also provides the patient and/or family members an opportunity to voice concerns and hopes about what the individual wants to achieve through therapy. This interchange between patient and therapist is extremely important in setting realistic short- and long-term goals and expectations. It is a process that will occur periodically as conditions change and goals are met. (See also Subjective Exam in Chapter 9.)

Cognition

Functions like orientation, attentiveness, long- and short-term memory, reasoning, and judgment can be impaired in disorders of the central nervous system and can have a major impact on the patient's ability to function in daily activities and return to school or work. If these impairments are present, they may be more thoroughly evaluated by a neuropsychologist, who can then also act as a resource for other team members regarding strategies to manage the problems. For example, patients with TBI often exhibit behavioral problems. To address these successfully, it is important that everyone in contact with the person respond similarly to these behaviors and give consistent responses. The specific strategies chosen would be determined by discussion among the team of care providers and the neuropsychologist, based on an evaluation and understanding of the underlying phenomena.

Communication

This is another area that will have a major impact on how the therapist works with the patient. If the patient exhibits a diminished ability to receive and interpret verbal or written communication **(receptive aphasia)** or an impaired ability to express herself/himself **(expressive aphasia),** then the therapist again will have to employ specific strategies to work with the patient successfully. For example, when working with patients with receptive aphasia, the therapist may need to physically mime or demonstrate to the patient what is expected or required and to use gestures to augment the words.

The objective evaluation continues, with the use of more traditional aspects of physical therapy. These are described below.

Functional Activities

The evaluation may begin with the therapist asking the patient to first demonstrate or describe activities and movements that the patient can perform and then describe activities that are difficult or that the patient is unable to perform. The most common activities of daily living (ADL) involve the ability to move and change positions in bed; to get in and out of bed, chair, etc.; to stand, walk, and climb stairs; and to get up from the floor in case of a fall. In short, these activities involve the ability to assume and maintain a posture and to function in different positions and environmental conditions. Several components are responsible for the smooth and efficient performance of even the simplest and most routine activities. A problem with even a single component can impair function.

Motor Control

The first component to examine in the evaluation of **motor control** is whether the patient is capable of performing voluntary, isolated activity of a specific muscle or whether the patient is only capable of performing movements that are linked together involuntarily. For example, very often in the early stages of recovery after a stroke, a patient is unable to isolate and restrict the activity of bringing the hand to the mouth without the automatic and involuntary activity of raising the shoulder. A second step is to determine whether the patient is able to isolate and *control* specific muscle activity and movements, (able to start, stop, reverse, change speed, direction, force, etc.) and if so, how well this is controlled. A third step is to determine whether the patient exhibits any involuntary movements. Do they occur at rest or with activity? Do the nature and intensity of the involuntary movements change with activity and are the movements detrimental to the patient's overall functioning? Finally, is the patient exhibiting any reflex reactions based on damage to specific parts of the nervous system? For example, when damage occurs to the cortex, the patient may exhibit certain reflexive reactions that are indicative of control exerted by the brainstem. These automatic reactions will prevent the patient from exerting independent and isolated control and thus affect function. (See also Chapter 7—Pediatric Physical Therapy.)

Tone

This is tension exerted and/or maintained by muscles at rest and during movement. In certain conditions, this **tone** is disturbed and a patient may exhibit **hypotonia** (low tone) or **hypertonia** (high tone). This disturbance of tone may be evident at rest and/or during activities. The following questions will need to be answered before making a decision regarding any interventions: Is the tone disturbance at a level which affects posture and function? What factors seem to increase or decrease it? Does it have a beneficial or detrimental effect on patient's ability to function?

Sensation and Perception

Both of these are essential for normal movement. **Sensation** is the ability to receive sensory input from within and outside the body and transmit it through the peripheral nerves and tracts in the spinal cord to the brain, where it is received and interpreted. Sensory information most essential for movement is visual, vestibular, tactile, and proprioceptive in nature. **Perception** is the ability to integrate various simultaneous sensory inputs and to respond appropriately. It is the latter ability that is most often affected in patients with brain lesions with a tremendous impact on movement and function.

Flexibility

The flexibility of the soft tissues, such as muscle and tendons, and the alignment and mobility of the joints are important to evaluate. Therapists perform manual tests and use goniometers to help quantify the degree of restriction of movement. (See Chapter 9—Orthopaedic Physical Therapy.)

From the above brief descriptions, it is apparent that movements and activities that seem so simple are the result of very complex and interconnected mechanisms. Sometimes it takes therapists several sessions to diagnose the movement disorders and identify the components that are responsible. Based on the findings of this completed, detailed evaluation, a treatment plan can be drawn up to meet the goal of enhancing movement and function.

TREATMENT
PRINCIPLES AND
TECHNIQUES

The human nervous system is an incredible system, capable of adaptation and modification after injury or disease, due to plasticity and redundancy. The peripheral nervous system also has the additional capacity for regeneration. Creative treatment approaches are necessary to accommodate these characteristics of the nervous system. This is the challenge and reward of working with patients with neurologic disorders.

Early approaches to neurological physical therapy focused on poliomyelitis. This disease causes paralysis of muscles due to damage to the motor nerve cells. It was one of the conditions responsible for the growth and development of physical therapy in the 1920s and 1930s.[10] As the poliomyelitis epidemics subsided, therapists started working with patients with other neurological conditions, such as stroke and cerebral palsy. As therapists worked with these patients, they found that treatments like hot packs, massage, stretching, and strengthening exercises—which had worked so well with the polio patients were not appropriate or sufficient for patients with other neurological problems. Therefore, between the 1940s and 1970s several therapists developed a variety of treatment and handling approaches based on their observations of motor behavior in their patients. They also found that they could influence the motor behavior with a variety of sensory inputs (e.g., visual, auditory, thermal, tactile, proprioceptive.) To understand and explain the phenomena they were observing, they turned to the literature available at the time. The work of neurophysiologists like Jackson, Sherrington, and Magnus provided some explanations and influenced treatment philosophies. These early approaches are briefly described.

Proprioceptive Neuromuscular Facilitation (PNF)

This is one of the earliest techniques developed by Dr. Kabat, a neurologist working with physical therapists Margaret Knott and Dorothy Voss. Working with patients with multiple sclerosis and cerebral palsy, Dr. Kabat observed that the "one muscle-one joint" approach used in the treatment of patients with polio was not applicable to this group. From his observations of normal human movement, he emphasized the fact that most human activities require multidimensional movements; that is, various muscles at various joints complement and enhance one another's activities. He also observed that motor performance could be facilitated and enhanced by providing the patient with sensory stimuli at specific locations and times within a movement.[10] Such techniques, as their name implies, emphasize proprioceptive (joint and position sense) stimuli, but also use tactile, visual, and auditory stimuli. These techniques are currently used to enhance movement and motor control not only in patients with neurological problems, but also in patients with musculoskeletal problems.

Rood's Approach

Margaret Rood recognized and emphasized the importance of sensory stimuli in arousing, calming, and modulating motor responses. She used a variety of stimuli to influence motor behavior. She also recognized and emphasized the importance of the autonomic nervous system in modulating motor responses.[13]

Brunnstrom's Approach

Signe Brunnstrom worked with patients who had suffered damage to the nervous system due to a CVA. She made detailed observations regarding the movement patterns these patients exhibited as they recovered. She was thus able to precisely describe the natural history of recovery of movement and function after a stroke. Based on her observations, as well as her extensive search and interpretation of the literature available, she made specific recommendations regarding the sequence of movements and activities that would facilitate recovery and function.[11] Her observations have been replicated, and her recommendations regarding treatment continue to be used.

Neurodevelopmental Treatment (NDT)

This approach was developed by Berta Bobath and Karel Bobath, her husband. Mrs. Bobath worked extensively with children with cerebral palsy and adult patients with stroke. Based on her observations in these patient populations and her interpretation of the works of Jackson, Sherrington, etc., she developed her theories and treatment approach. Her hypothesis, especially in regard to adult patients with stroke, asserts that because of the damage caused by the stroke, the patient is unable to direct the nervous impulses appropriately.[3] This results in abnormal patterns of coordination in posture and movement and in abnormal qualities of tone.[11] The aim of treatment is to inhibit the abnormal patterns of movement and facilitate integrated, automatic reactions and voluntary functional activity.

Techniques based on all these approaches continue to be used to improve motor control. Their efficacy is still being established and researched. No specific technique has been proven to be more effective than others, and therapists continue to mix and match them based on patient needs.

Current Approaches

Over the past 20 years our understanding of motor development, motor control, and **motor learning** has increased tremendously. This has led to a review and re-evaluation of the earlier techniques—those that emphasized inhibitory and facilitatory inputs and modifying motor behavior through handling.[15] Based on the principles of motor learning and skill acquisition, current approaches put less emphasis on passive handling of the patient.[6] They recommend a more active involvement on the part of the patient, especially in terms of problem solving and finding appropriate solutions.[5] They emphasize the need for the therapist to create the appropriate environment for learning and the appropriate use of feedback to facilitate learning.

Besides these specific techniques, therapists may choose options that are specifically targeted to the impairments and dysfunction. These techniques include stretching or strengthening exercises to improve flexibility and strength. Other options may be more compensatory or adaptive. For instance, the therapist may teach a patient with impaired sensation in the soles of the feet to rely more on the eyes and visual system for maintenance of balance; another may initiate the use of braces to improve walking in the case of irreversible paralysis of leg muscles. The therapist may also recommend environmental modifications to help the patient function better. Thus a therapist is constantly challenged to be as creative as possible in treating and managing the movement-related problems of function due to disorders of the nervous system.

CASE STUDY

Jim is an eighteen-year-old male who sustained a gun shot wound to his thoracic spine. The shot ruptured his spine, causing damage to the spinal cord which resulted in paralysis below the waist. He also sustained abdominal injuries that required surgery. He is now medically stable and referred to therapy to begin the long process of rehabilitation.

The first task of the team members (which include a physiatrist, nurse, psychologist, social worker, and physical and occupational therapists) is to complete detailed evaluations. This may take several days because each team member is working within the constraints imposed by the patient's physical and emotional condition. When all the information is gathered, a team meeting is scheduled to discuss the information with the patient and his family and to start setting some short- and long-term goals.

Even as they were carrying out their evaluations, the team members had already started treatment and management to maintain mobility, increase strength in uninvolved muscles, and educate the patient about problems arising from loss of sensation. The nurses had initiated a program to manage bowel and bladder function. The psychologist had begun helping Jim cope with the trauma of this unexpected event and the loss of body image and body functions. The social worker was starting to determine Jim's needs upon discharge and whether these needs could be met by his family and in the current home environment.

During the next several weeks, the physicians will continue to check Jim thoroughly to see if there is any change or return of sensory or motor activity because that will determine the final prognosis. Other team members will continue to work with Jim to teach the new skills necessary to function within the new reality. The physical therapist will play a major role in teaching and training him in these new skills. The therapist will also be involved in ordering equipment like the appropriate wheelchair, cushion, etc., to meet the needs of his lifestyle. The therapist will make recommendations to the family for a ramp to gain access to the house. The family may need to widen doorways and remove carpeting to make wheelchair mobility and access easier. They made need to adapt/build a bathroom and bedroom on the main floor level to meet Jim's needs. They may be able to get some financial help or they may end up bearing the complete financial burden themselves.

Not only is their son dealing with a lot of physical and psychological challenges, but also the family is dealing with a lot of emotional issues. As the therapist trains the family to assist Jim, very often during these sessions family members will be very open, voicing their fears and concerns. The therapist's role then is to provide not only technical support for the physical needs, but also psychological and emotional support to both the patient and the family.

SUMMARY

The goal of neurologic physical therapy is to treat problems of movement and function that result from damage to the nervous system. If the problems are untreatable and progressive, the goal is to teach the patient and caregivers to accommodate and compensate for the problems and prevent secondary complications. To achieve these goals, the therapists need to evaluate the components necessary for movement and assess their role in the dysfunction. Based on the findings, the therapist—in conjunction with the patient, family, and other caregivers—will draw up a plan of care with appropriate short- and long-term goals and specific strategies to meet those goals. This process of evaluation, assessment, and treatment will occur periodically as goals are met. If goals become unachievable due to physical, psychological, or social factors, a re-evaluation of goals and strategies becomes necessary.

The ultimate objective is to help rehabilitate the patient so that he or she can function at the highest level of ability attainable.

References

1. Adams RD, Victor M: Special techniques for neurologic diagnosis. In Adams RD, Victor M: Principles of neurology, New York, 1989, McGraw Hill.

2. Bannister R: Parkinsonism and movement disorders. In Bannister R: Brain and Bannister's Clinical Nuerology, Oxford, England, 1992, Oxford Medical Publications.

3. Bobath B: Adult hemiplegia: evaluation and treatment, Oxford, England, 1990, Butterworth Heinemann.

4. Brooke M: Diseases of the motor neurons. In Brooke M: A clinicians view of neuromuscular diseases, Baltimore, 1986, Williams and Wilkins.

5. Carr JH, Shepherd RB: A motor relearning program for stroke, Rockville, 1987, Aspen Publishers.

6. Carr JH, Shepherd RB: Movement science, foundation for physical therapy in rehabilitation, Rockville, 1987, Aspen Publishers.

7. Leahy P: Traumatic head injury. In O'Sullivan SB, Schmitz TJ, editors: Physical rehabilitation assessment and treatment, Philadelphia, 1994, F. A. Davis Co.

8. O'Sullivan SB: Multiple sclerosis, In O'Sullivan SB, Schmitz TJ, editors: Physical rehabilitation assessment and treatment, Philadelphia, 1994, F. A. Davis Co.

9. O'Sullivan SB: Stroke. In O'Sullivan SB, Schmitz TJ, editors: Physical rehabilitation assessment and treatment, Philadelphia, 1994, F. A. Davis Co.

10. Pinkston D: Evolution of the practice of physical therapy in the united states. In Scully RM, Barnes MR, editors: Physical therapy, Philadelphia, 1989, JB Lippincott Co.

11. Sawner K, Lavigne J: Brunnstrom's movement therapy in hemiplegia, Philadelphia, 1992, JB Lippincott Co.

12. Schmitz TJ: Traumatic spinal cord injury. In O'Sullivan SB, Schmitz TJ, editors: Physical rehabilitation assessment and treatment, Philadelphia, 1994, F. A. Davis Co.

13. Stockmeyer SA: An interpretation of approach of Rood to the treatment of neuromuscular dysfunction, In Bouman HD, editor: Proceedings: An exploratory and analytical survey of therapeutic exercise, Am J Phy Med 46(1):900-956, 1967.

14. Voss DE, Ionta MK, Myers BJ, et al: Proprioceptive neuromuscular facilitation, ed 3, Philadelphia, 1985, Harper and Row.

15. Umphred DN: Merging neurophysiologic approaches with contemporary theories. In Lister MJ, editor: Contemporary management of motor control problems, Alexandria, VA, 1991, Foundation for Physical Therapy.

Suggested Readings

The following is a list of books published for patients and their families to gain a better understanding of causes, clinical features, diagnostic procedures, treatment and management principles and the role of the various team members in caring for patients with the noted disorders.

Caroscio JT, editor: Amyotrophic lateral sclerosis: a guide for Patient Care, New York, 1986, Thieme Medical Publishers.

Duvoisin RC, editor: Parkinson's disease: a guide for patients and their families, ed 3, New York, 1991 Raven Press.

Faye-Pierson J, Toole JF, editors: Stroke: a guide for patients and their families, New York, 1987, Raven Press.

Philips L, et al, editors: Spinal cord injury: a guide for patients and their families, New York, 1987, Raven Press.

Ringel SP, editor: Neuromuscular disorders: a guide for patient care, New York, 1987, Raven Press.

Schienberg LC, editor: Multiple sclerosis: a guide for patients and their families, New York, 1983, Raven Press.

Umphred DN: Neurological rehabilitation, ed 3, St. Louis, Mosby-Year Book. A comprehensive text on the rehabilitation of patients with neurological disorders, including the pediatric and adult populations. Recommended for upper division students and as a reference for practicing therapists/assistants interested in neurological disorders. A student workbook is also available.

Review Questions

1. Why might the physical therapy treatment plan change several times for a patient recovering from a stroke?

2. What function do bone grafts, rods, wires, body jackets and casts play in neurological rehabilitation? Briefly discuss other devices used in neurological rehabilitation.

3. Contrast the differing roles the physical therapist and physical therapist assistant may assume, depending on the nature of the patient's neurologic condition (e.g., contrast physical therapist's roles for patients with the following: spinal cord injury, stroke, Parkinson's disease, and ALS).

4. Describe the main differences between purposes of at least three diagnostic tests in neurological disorders. How do they differ in procedure as well?

5. Make a list of the kinds of information you might hope to gain from interviewing the patient and family, particularly in neurological rehabilitation.

6. Why is it a concern if a patient who performs multidimensional tasks can't isolate a much simpler movement?

7. Contrast and compare three different treatment approaches discussed in this chapter.

Chapter 9

Orthopaedic Physical Therapy

Barbara C. Belyea
Hilary B. Greenberger

"The weakest link in a chain is the strongest because it can break it."
Stanislaw J. Lec

KEY TERMS

accessory motion of the joint
active-assisted ROM
active-free ROM
active range of motion (AROM)
active-resisted exercises
aerobics training
bursitis
closed chain exercise/kinetic chain exercise
cryotherapy
dysfunction
electrical stimulation
flexibility
flexibility exercise
fluidotherapy
functional exercises
goniometer
goniometry

hot packs
hydrotherapy
hypermobile joint
hypomobile joint
infrared
joint mobilization
manual muscle testing (MMT)
massage
muscle endurance
muscular strength
myofascial release
nerve entrapment
objective examination
open chain exercises/joint isolation exercises
paraffin treatment
passive range of motion (PROM)
proprioception
proprioceptors
range-of-motion exercise
resisted exercise
resisted test
short wave diathermy
soft tissue mobilizations
special tests
sprain
strain
strength
subjective evaluation
tendinitis
thermal agents
ultrasound
whirlpools

One of the largest clinical specialties within the physical therapy profession, orthopaedic physical therapy encompasses a wide array of therapeutic techniques and philosophies of treatment. Physical therapists practicing in the field of orthopaedics work in a variety of clinical settings and treat patients of diverse ages who present with a variety of physical and medical problems. This chapter will describe the types of patients treated by an orthopaedic physical therapist and present some of the evaluation techniques and treatment approaches commonly used.

GENERAL
DESCRIPTION

While the clinical interests or approaches to treatment may be diverse, the common thread throughout orthopaedic physical therapy is the focus on a patient's function. Through an evaluation process, the orthopaedic therapist assesses the cause and extent of any functional disability, referred to as a **"dysfunction,"** and works with the patient to return the individual to an optimal level of function. A person's function can be affected when a disruption occurs in the musculoskeletal system, either due to a traumatic injury or from repeated stress to tissue. Dysfunctions may be caused by a structural imbalance either of muscle or bone, birth defects, results of surgery, or degenerative changes in the body.[12] Dysfunctions of the musculoskeletal system often result in symptoms of pain, stiffness, edema (swelling), muscle weakness or fatigue, or loss of range of motion (movement at a joint).

In order to conduct a comprehensive evaluation and develop an appropriate treatment plan, therapists must have an extensive understanding of anatomy, biomechanics, pathokinesiology, exercise physiology, and the application of various treatment techniques. They must also be able to analyze clinical situations and problem-solve in order to determine which approach is the most appropriate for each patient situation. Finally, it is also critical for therapists to have effective communication skills in order to establish good rapport with patients and to provide the necessary information to gain the patient's compliance with the treatment plan.

Development

The field of orthopaedic physical therapy has experienced significant growth in recent years for several reasons. Perhaps the most positive is the development of both sophisticated medical technology and new treatment techniques. Changes in lifestyle have also contributed to the growth of orthopaedic physical therapy. The population's increasing interest and participation in physical fitness has resulted in an increase in musculoskeletal dysfunctions due to overuse or traumatic injuries. The increased use of computers and other technical machinery requiring repeated motions has also had an impact in the incidence of overuse injuries in the upper extremity. Individuals who must sustain postures at a computer or machinery while performing repeated motions with their hands may develop muscle injury or nerve entrapment that require intervention by a physical therapist. An increase in life span has also resulted in the growth of this area of physical therapy as people are living longer and experiencing symptoms related to degenerative changes in their bodies.

A great deal of similarity exists between orthopaedic physical therapy and sports physical therapy. In both areas, the focus of physical therapy is to regain optimum function and return the patient to the previous level of function and activity. For the sports physical therapist, this means incorporating sport-specific activities into the treatment program to make sure the patient can meet the physical demands of the sport with respect to strength, endurance, balance, and speed. The orthopaedic physical therapist may work with athletes, but may also treat a variety of musculoskeletal conditions that are not related to sports activities.

COMMON
CONDITIONS

Within the broad scope of orthopaedic physical therapy, a variety of patient problems may be treated. These conditions range from injuries sustained through athletic participation, work-related injuries, dysfunction following orthopaedic surgical procedures, or the degenerative changes that accompany the aging process. As previously stated, patients referred to physical therapy with orthopaedic conditions may present with pain, swelling, weakness, or loss of motion resulting from trauma to the musculoskeletal system. This includes damage to bones or soft tissues such as muscles, tendons, joint capsules, ligaments, bursae, and fascia in the extremities or spine.

Injuries to joints or soft tissues may be the result of either repeated stress or traumatic injury. Repeated stress to an area of the body can cause overuse injuries, which may result in inflammation of soft tissue. The following examples describe some common conditions caused by overuse injuries.

Overuse Injuries

Bursitis. Bursitis is an inflammation of bursae, which are fluid-filled sacs located throughout the body that serve to decrease the friction between two structures. Bursae become irritated and painful when they are repeatedly pinched between two structures. A common example of this occurs at the shoulder, when the subacromial bursa gets pinched during repeated movements when the shoulder is in an overhead position, as with painting, reaching or throwing motions.

Tendinitis. Tendinitis is an inflammation of a tendon, which is a structure located at the ends of muscles and that attaches muscles to bone. Repeated use of muscles can cause stress to the tendon and result in painful movement. Tendinitis is frequently seen in the patellar tendon at the knee in people who perform repeated jumping (e.g., dancers, basketball players) and at the elbow in people who do repeated or sustained gripping activities (e.g., carpenters, tennis players).

Nerve Entrapment. Pressure on a nerve may result from a variety of sources, and usually causes symptoms of tingling, pain, and/or weakness. A common condition of nerve compression at the wrist is referred to as carpal tunnel syndrome. Patients with carpal tunnel syndrome usually complain of numbness and pain in the hand and fingers, commonly resulting from repeated activities with the wrist in a flexed position (e.g., musicians, computer keyboard operators).

Traumatic Injuries

In contrast to overuse injuries, musculoskeletal injuries may also occur as the result of direct trauma. Bones, muscles, ligaments, and other soft tissue may be injured when they sustain a direct blow, or when they are placed under excessive stretch. The following examples are just a few of the common conditions that can arise from direct trauma to the musculoskeletal system.

Ligament Sprain. Ligaments are supporting structures at joints that serve to stabilize the joint and prevent excess movement. When ligaments are overstretched, their fibers can tear, causing pain and instability at the joint. A common site of **sprain** is at the ankle when the lateral (outside) ligaments are overstretched. This occurs when a person lands on the foot in a turned-in position. Another common site of ligament sprain is the anterior cruciate ligament (ACL) at the knee. Injuries to the ACL are usually the result of a twisting movement when the foot is planted, as seen with quick turns during running.

Fracture. Direct trauma to bone can result in a break, or fracture of the bone. Fractures can occur at any bone in the body, but are commonly seen at the wrist or the hip following falls. Elderly individuals are particularly prone to fractures due to changes in the structure of their bones resulting from inactivity, inadequate nutrition, and degenerative changes. Fractures are best diagnosed through the use of radiographs.

Muscle Strain. A sudden contraction of a muscle or excessive stretch to a muscle can cause tearing of the muscle fibers, known as a **strain.** Muscle strains can occur in any area of the body, and can range in severity. Low back strains can occur during improper lifting techniques, and cervical strains may be the result of a sudden movement of the neck, as with a whiplash injury. A complete rupture of the muscle may be seen in the ankle (Achilles rupture) or elbow (biceps rupture) and must be surgically repaired.

Surgical Conditions

Individuals who have had surgery are another group of patients commonly seen by the orthopaedic physical therapist. Injuries resulting from either repeated stress, acute trauma, or disease processes may require surgical intervention for appropriate healing. The following are examples of orthopaedic surgeries that can benefit from physical therapy intervention to reduce pain and regain motion and strength in order to allow for optimal movement and function.

Total Joint Replacement. Degenerative changes at joint surfaces, causing painful movement, can be alleviated through surgical replacement of the joint surfaces. Joints most commonly replaced are weight-bearing joints, primarily hips and knees. A variety of plastic and stainless steel implants are used to effectively replace degenerated joint surfaces. Therapeutic intervention is necessary post-operatively to ensure maximum strength and function, and to prevent complications, such as a dislocation.

Amputation. A surgical amputation is the removal of a portion of an extremity either due to trauma, inadequate blood flow or the presence of a malignant growth. Inadequate circulation can be the result of disease processes such as diabetes mellitus or peripheral vascular disease, while a growth may indicate the presence of cancer.

Medical Conditions

Other medical conditions may also affect the musculoskeletal system by causing weakness or loss of function. Systemic diseases such as rheumatoid arthritis, cancer, or Acquired Immunodeficiency Syndrome (AIDS) may produce weakness or functional challenges that can be addressed by the orthopaedic physical therapist.

EVALUATION PRINCIPLES AND TECHNIQUES

Treating a patient with a musculoskeletal injury requires the physical therapist to have an understanding of the injury in order to provide appropriate treatment. This understanding is accomplished by completing an initial evaluation—that is, a thorough evaluation of the patient on the initial visit. Subsequent re-evaluations are performed throughout the rehabilitative process in order to monitor patient progress.

This section will discuss the following components of an initial evaluation: patient history, observation, active and passive range of motion, strength, flexibility, functional assessments/tests, special tests, palpation, and other diagnostic procedures. The first activity is part of the subjective exam, whereas the remaining ones comprise the objective exam.

Subjective Exam

Interviewing the patient about the extent and nature of an injury is referred to as the **subjective evaluation.** It is a qualitative measurement based on the *patient's* perception of the problem. It is therefore included in the "S" portion of the "SOAP" note (See Chapter 2).

The role of the therapist during the interview is to guide the patient through pertinent questions. This interaction allows the therapist to develop a rapport with the patient and to understand the patient's insight into and opinion of the problem. The interview also assists the therapist in appropriately directing the remainder of the evaluation. Often, the patient interview will give the therapist ample information to make a tentative physical therapy diagnosis. Questions asked during the interview include information on the cause of the injury, current symptoms, previous physical therapy treatments, past medical history, and lifestyle as it pertains to work and recreation. Box 9-1 lists typical questions asked during the patient interview.

Box 9-1

Questions typically asked during the subjective component of an initial physical therapy evaluation

1. What brings you to physical therapy today?

2. What do you feel is your primary problem? Is it stiffness? Pain?

3. Was the onset of the problem slow or sudden? Was there a mechanism of injury?

4. Have you ever had this problem before? If so, were you treated for it? How long did it take to recover?

5. What provokes your symptoms? What relieves your symptoms?

6. Are your symptoms worsening or improving?

7. Are your symptoms constant or intermittent?

8. Can you describe your pain? Does your pain spread to other parts of your body?

9. What is your occupation?

10. Have you had any radiographs ("x-rays") taken?

11. Are you currently taking any medication for this problem?

12. Is there anything else you would like to tell me that I have not asked that would be pertinent to your problem?

Frequently, the patient will be asked to draw the location of the pain on a body chart (Fig. 9-1). Pain scales are also often used to gauge the amount of pain that the patient is experiencing (Fig. 9-2). Following the interview, and prior to the objective evaluation, the therapist should have gained information regarding the location of pain, nature of the disorder (acute versus chronic condition) and behavior of the symptoms (what activities make the symptoms either better or worse).

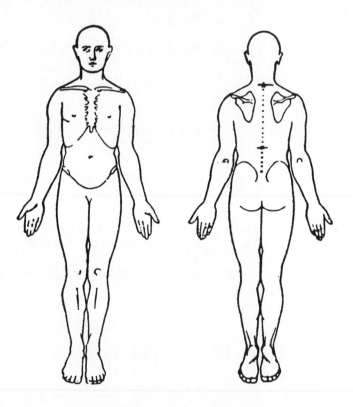

Fig. 9-1. Body Chart to indicate area(s) of pain. Patient is asked to indicate area(s) of pain with XXX; area(s) of numbness with ///; area(s) of tingling with +++.

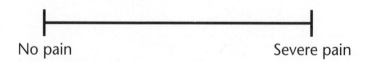

No pain   Severe pain

Fig. 9-2. Visual Analog Scale (VAS). On the line provided, patient is asked to mark the degree of pain experienced.

Objective Exam

The **objective examination** refers to quantitative or qualitative measurements that are taken by the *physical therapist.* Specific numbers or grades may be assigned (quantitative measurement), as is the case with range of motion measurements or strength measurements. Other times, parts of the evaluation are performed by observing and describing patterns of movement and/or deformities (qualitative measurement). The information derived from this portion of the examination is included in the "O" section of the SOAP note (See Chapter 2). The purpose of the objective examination is to establish baseline values and observations that can be used as a comparison following a single treatment or a series of treatments. This allows the physical therapist to make appropriate changes in the treatment plan based on the amount of progress or lack of progress found during the objective exam.

This section will briefly describe the various aspects of the objective examination. The purpose is for the introductory level student to become familiar with common terms used when working with a patient who has an orthopaedic problem.

Observation. Observation is the "looking" phase of the examination. It may begin in the waiting room where the therapist can observe the general attitude of the patient, general posture, and willingness to move. A perfunctory gait assessment may be made as the patient enters the evaluation area. Once the patient is appropriately undressed, a more detailed inspection can be made. This may include observing obvious deformities such as a curvature in the spine, joint subluxations (a condition where a joint partially dislocates), asymmetrical body contours, swelling, and color and texture of the skin. Many musculoskeletal injuries are a result of or exacerbated by poor sitting and standing postures. Therefore, particular attention is paid to the standing and sitting posture of the patient.

Active Range of Motion. Active range of motion (AROM) refers to the ability of the *patient* to *voluntarily* move a limb through an arc of movement. Active range of motion provides the therapist with information regarding the quality of the movement (smooth versus rigid movement), the willingness of the patient to move the limb, the pain produced during movement, and whether there are any limitations in the motion as compared to the unaffected side. An example of AROM of the shoulder in multiple planes is provided in Fig. 9-3.

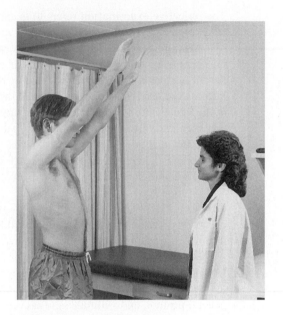

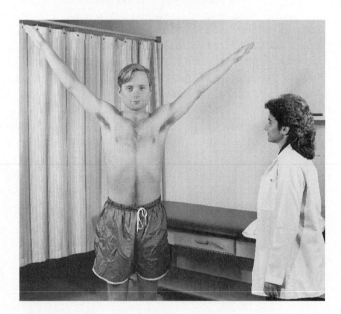

Fig. 9-3. Examination of active range of motion at the shoulder. **A.** Shoulder flexion. **B.** Shoulder abduction. (Photo credits: Dewey Neild).

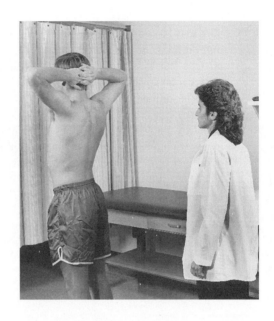

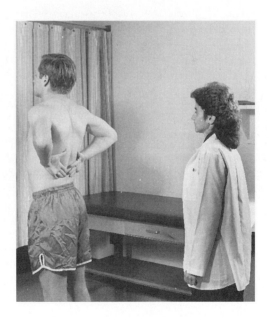

Fig. 9-3. Examination of active range of motion at the shoulder. **C.** Shoulder external rotation. **D.** Shoulder internal rotation. (Photo credits: Dewey Neild).

Passive Range of Motion. Passive range of motion (PROM) refers to the amount of movement at a joint that is obtained by the *therapist* moving the segment *without assistance from the patient.* In some instances, due to injury or prolonged immobilization, a joint may have less motion than is considered functional. This is referred to as a **hypomobile joint.** In other cases, such as a subluxing joint, the joint may have excessive motion. This is referred to as a **hypermobile joint.** Passive range of motion will also give the therapist an indication of the degree and pattern of pain, as well as the "feel" of the movement.

There are many methods to measure and document PROM. The most common measurement technique is called **goniometry** and is performed using a **goniometer.** Examples of different types of goniometers are illustrated in Fig. 9-4. The amount of motion available at any joint is dependent on the structure of the joint. Additionally, norm values for joint range of motion are dependent on several factors including the age and gender of the patient.[3] Typically, a therapist will compare range of motion values of the affected joint to that of the unaffected side. Fig. 9-5 is an example of a physical therapist conducting a PROM measurement of a patient's knee flexion.

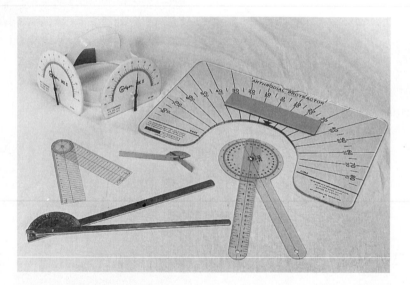

Fig. 9-4. Variety of goniometers to measure joint angles. Size and type vary to measure long and short limb segments, and cervical region (Photo credit: Dewey Neild).

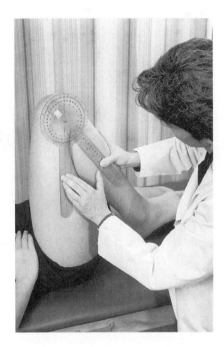

Fig. 9-5. Physical therapist conducting a goniometric measurement of knee flexion (Photo credit: Dewey Neild).

Strength. Strength can be defined as the amount of force produced during a voluntary muscular contraction. This contraction may be performed statically (no motion) or dynamically (through a range of motion). When assessing the status of the muscles and tendons, a quick **resisted test** is used. This allows the therapist to determine the general strength of a muscle group and assess whether any pain is produced with the muscle contraction.

If it is determined from the resisted test that a muscle or muscle group is weak or painful, then further testing is performed to isolate the specific muscle. To isolate and test specific muscles, **manual muscle testing (MMT)** is performed (Fig. 9-6). Manual muscle testing allows the therapist to assign a specific grade to a muscle. This grade is based on whether the patient can hold the limb against gravity, how much manual resistance can be tolerated, and whether there is full range of motion at a joint. There are several systems of grading that are widely used. One of the most common grading systems was initially described by Robert Lovett, MD and later modified by Henry Kendall, PT, and Florence Kendall, PT.[7] This key to muscle grading is outlined in Table 9-1.

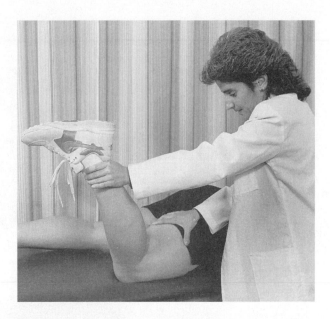

Fig. 9-6. Physical therapists commonly perform manual muscle tests to determine muscle strength. Pictured is the manual muscle test for the hamstring musculature. (Photo credit: Dewey Neild).

With the advent of highly technological equipment, there are now many other sophisticated methods to measure strength. This includes computerized instruments such as isokinetic devices. These machines allow the therapist to obtain strength curves of isolated muscles as well as specific force values. These machines will be discussed in more detail in the treatment section of this chapter.

Flexibility. Flexibility refers to the ability to move a limb segment through a range of motion. The amount of flexibility an individual has at a given joint depends on a combination of two factors. First, the soft tissue surrounding the joint must be pliable to allow movement between the joint surfaces. This is referred to as **accessory motion of the joint.** Accessory motion refers to the ability of the joint surfaces to glide, roll, and spin on each other. Secondly, the muscle or muscles crossing the joint must be at an appropriate length to allow motion to occur. For example, the ability to stand up and reach to touch your toes while keeping your knees straight would depend on the flexibility of the back and posterior hip muscles, as well as the ability of the spinal vertebrae to move.

Table 9-1. Key to Manual Muscle Testing Grades*

	Function of the muscle	Grade	Symbols	
No Movement	No contraction felt in the muscle	Zero	0	0
	Tendon becomes prominent or feeble contraction felt in the muscle, but no visible movement of the part	Trace	T	1
Test Movement	**MOVEMENT IN HORIZONTAL PLANE**			
	Moves through partial range of motion	Poor-	P-	2-
	Moves through complete range of motion	Poor	P	2
	Moves to completion of range against resistance or moves to completion of range against pressure	Poor+	P+	2+
	ANTIGRAVITY POSITION			
	Moves through partial range of motion			
Test Position	Gradual release from test position	Fair-	F-	3-
	Holds test position (no added pressure)	Fair	F	3
	Holds test position against slight pressure	Fair+	F+	3+
	Holds test position against slight to moderate pressure	Good-	G-	4-
	Holds test position against moderate pressure	Good	G	4
	Holds test position against moderate to strong pressure	Good+	G+	4+
	Holds test position against strong pressure	Normal	N	5

* 1993 Florence P. Kendall. Modified from Kendall FP, McCreary EK, Provance PG: Muscles Testing and Function, 4, Baltimore, 1993, Williams & Wilkins, page 189. Author grants permission to reproduce this chart.

Appropriate flexibility or balance of muscles is a key component to proper posture and body mechanics. Almost all of the musculoskeletal problems seen in the physical therapy clinic can be linked to muscle imbalances. For example, if the muscles surrounding the shoulder did not act synergistically (due to a lack of flexibility), this may cause a compensation at joints distal and proximal to the shoulder, such as the elbow and cervical spine.

There are many tests that a physical therapist may perform to determine flexibility. One common test for the lower extremity is called the 90/90 straight leg raise (Fig. 9-7). This test objectively measures hamstring flexibility, the muscle on the posterior aspect of the thigh.

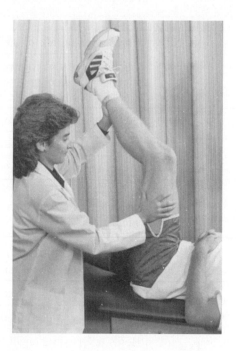

Fig. 9-7. Example of a test for flexibility: the 90/90 straight leg raise (Photo credit: Dewey Neild).

Functional Assessments/Tests. The ultimate goal in therapy is to return the patient to his or her prior level of activity. This may include anything from the ability to go grocery shopping independently to returning to athletic competition. In some types of injuries, returning to prior level of activity is not feasible. In these cases, the ultimate goal would be to return the individual to his or her highest level of function achievable.

Traditionally, when we think of functional assessments, we refer to activities such as the patient's bed mobility; transferring between a variety of surfaces (e.g., moving from a sitting position in a wheelchair to a standing position); and the ability to perform activities of daily living (ADLs) such as combing hair, dressing, and bathing. Physical therapists may spend a large percentage of their time during the initial evaluation assessing the patient's ability to perform these ADLs. This becomes particularly important when working with patients who are post-surgical. An example would be a patient who is seen following a total joint replacement of the hip or knee. Box 9-2 lists examples of ADLs.

Box 9-2

Examples of Activities of Daily Living

Eating
- eat with spoon
- eat with fork
- cut with knife
- open milk carton
- pour liquid
- drink from cup

Dressing and Undressing
- reach clothes in closet
- put on shoe
- manage zippers
- remove coat

Bathing/Grooming
- turn on faucet
- wash hands
- dry with towel
- manage cosmetics
- brush teeth

Bed/Bathroom
- get out of bed
- transfer to toilet
- reach objects on nightstand
- sit up in bed

Transfer/Ambulatory Activities
- in and out of bus
- in and out of car
- safe outdoor ambulation
- endurance

Other Activities
- propel wheelchair forwards
- propel wheelchair backwards
- manage elevator
- hold book
- dial a telephone
- use scissors

Recently, there has been a surge of literature in the orthopaedic and sports physical therapy arena regarding the importance of functional testing for individuals returning to activities other than ADLs.[1,2,9,13] These activities may include sports, gait, lifting tasks, and other multiplanar movements. Examples of functional tests for these activities include hop tests, jump tests, lunge tests, excursion tests, and balance tests. Gray has described these tests in detail.[6]

Special Tests. Special tests are used to evaluate specific joints to indicate the presence or absence of a particular problem. The purpose of these tests is to confirm and/or reinforce a physical therapy diagnosis. Because there are so many special tests available at each joint, only those that appear to be indicated, based on the results of the evaluation, are performed. Examples of special tests include those that examine nerve compression (Phalen's test, Fig. 9-8A); tests for shoulder impingement (Hawkin's test, Fig. 9-8B); and tests for ligamentous knee injuries (Lachman's test, Fig. 9-8C).

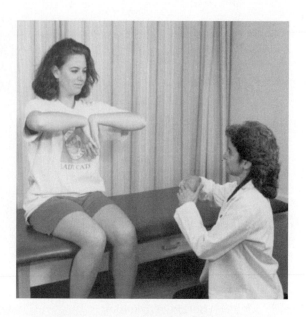

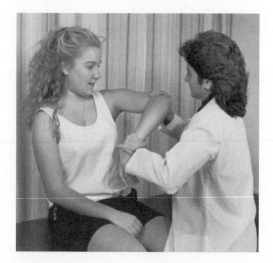

Fig. 9-8. Examples of special tests. **A.** Phalen's test for nerve compression. **B.** Hawkin's test for shoulder impingement. (Photo credits: Dewey Neild).

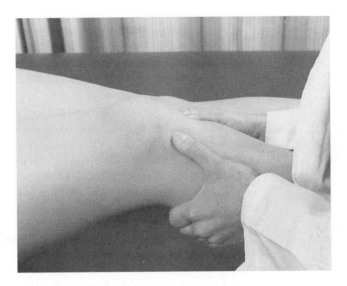

Fig. 9-8. Examples of special tests. **C.** Lachman's test for anterior cruciate ligament instability. (Photo credits: Dewey Neild).

Palpation. A comprehensive understanding of anatomy is essential for any physical therapist. In the clinical situation, the therapist uses the sense of touch, known as palpation, to assess what is occurring below the skin and what musculoskeletal structures are involved with an injury. When palpating an area of the body, the therapist is feeling for areas of pain and tenderness, areas of restriction, swelling, and whether structures are properly oriented.

Other Diagnostic Procedures. Depending on the patient's injury or complaint, other evaluative procedures may be performed to provide a more complete assessment of the patient. The patient may be referred to other personnel for these procedures. This may include a variety of imaging techniques such as radiographs, computerized axial tomography scans (CAT scans); and magnetic resonance imaging (MRI). If the patient has had neurological damage, full sensory testing may be indicated. Additional tests for cardiopulmonary patients may include an assessment of lung capacity. Some of these tests are presented in more detail in Chapters 8 and 10.

Based on the interpretation of the findings from the comprehensive evaluation, the physical therapist identifies the limitations a patient has and determines the probable source of the problem. As previously stated, most patients with orthopaedic dysfunctions report symptoms of pain, loss of motion or strength, or edema. Once the problems have been identified, the therapist and patient develop goals to address each problem. Common goals are to decrease pain, decrease edema, increase strength, or increase motion. The ultimate goal for patients with orthopaedic dysfunctions is to achieve an optimal level of function, whether that means returning to work, returning to the athletic field, or resuming the ability to perform daily activities independently. Therapeutic goals should include the anticipated return of strength or function, and the expected time frame for rehabilitation. Once goals have been established, the therapist then develops a treatment plan designed to achieve these goals.

TREATMENT PRINCIPLES AND TECHNIQUES

Treatment planning is based on determining what intervention will most effectively improve a patient's function by decreasing pain, decreasing edema, increasing strength, or increasing motion. The treatment options and rehabilitation approaches available to the orthopaedic physical therapist are numerous. Some therapists may focus their treatment approaches on exercises, while others may incorporate physical agents or manual techniques. In most instances, a combination of techniques is most appropriate when designing a comprehensive plan to address the needs of the orthopaedic patient. Whatever approach is selected, the most important factor to consider when planning the treatment is to consider the goals of treatment and the goals of the patient.

The following discussion of treatment options is meant to introduce the reader to the typical indications and uses of various treatment techniques. The techniques described include: physical agents, manual techniques (including soft tissue and joint mobilization) and therapeutic exercise. The reader is referred to the reading list at the end of the chapter for sources which provide in-depth information regarding the application of these techniques.

Physical Agents

Many therapeutic agents are available for physical therapists to incorporate into orthopaedic rehabilitation programs. Based on the intended purpose and method of application, physical agents can be divided into two categories: thermal agents (thermotherapy) and electrical stimulation (electrotherapy). Thermal agents can be subdivided into agents that apply superficial heat, deep heat, and cold. The decision as to which agent to use is based on a thorough evaluation of the patient's symptoms, the goals of therapy, and the therapist's knowledge of the physiological and clinical effects of each physical agent. Table 9-2 lists the common physical agents used in physical therapy according to their *physical* effects and includes their *physiological* effects and clinical indications.

Thermal Agents. When a tissue in the body sustains an injury, an automatic response is initiated in an attempt to heal the tissue and return it to its pre-injured state. These naturally occurring processes are referred to as inflammation and repair.[14] The inflammation and repair stages of tissue healing can be altered through the use of thermal agents or electrotherapy. **Thermal agents** are used to modify the temperature of surrounding tissue and result in a change in the amount of blood flow to the injured area. In addition to vascular changes, temperature changes also have an effect on the metabolism of the surrounding tissue, as well as altering the neuromuscular and connective tissue. Through the use of therapeutic changes in temperature, the healing process can be accelerated and the injured tissue restored to optimal strength and integrity.

Table 9-2. Summary of Common Physical Agents Used in Physical Therapy

Physical Effect	Physical Agents	Physiological Effects	Clinical Indications
Superficial Heat	Hot packs Infrared Paraffin Fluidotherapy Whirlpool	Increases blood flow Increases metabolism: promotes healing and removal of waste products Decreases pain Decreases stiffness	Muscle spasm Pain Joint stiffness Wound care
Deep Heat	Ultrasound Short-wave diathermy	Increases blood flow Increases metabolism: promotes healing and removal of waste products Decreases pain Decreases stiffness	Muscle spasm Pain Joint stiffness
Cold	Ice packs Ice massage Cold whirlpool Cold compression	Decreases blood flow Decreases metabolism Decreases edema Decreases pain	Acute injury Swelling Pain Muscle spasm Post-exercise
Electrical Simulation	Transcutaneous Electrical Nerve Stimulation (TENS) Iontophoresis Electrical Stimulation for Tissue Repair (ESTR) Neuromuscular Electrical Stimulation (NMES)	Decreases pain Decreases edema Promotes wound healing Muscle reeducation Decreases spasticity	Pain Edema Wounds Nerve regeneration Muscle weakness/ imbalance

The extent of therapeutic changes caused by a change in tissue temperature depends on the intensity of the thermal agent applied, the length of time the tissue is exposed to the agent, and characteristics of the tissue being treated. The therapist must continually monitor and re-evaluate the patient to ensure that the thermal agent selected is appropriate and that the treatment goals are being achieved.

Thermal agents can be classified as those that provide superficial heat, deep heat, or cold. Superficial heat modalities create an increase in the blood flow to cutaneous tissues close to the surface, thereby reducing pain, reducing muscle spasm, allowing for increased motion, and promoting healing.[11] Examples of superficial heat agents include: hot packs, infrared, paraffin, fluidotherapy, and whirlpools.

Hot packs are pouches of various shapes that are filled with silica gel and soaked in thermostatically controlled water (Fig. 9-9). Hot packs are applied to the affected body part with layers of towels to prevent overheating (See Fig. 2-10 in Chapter 2). Similar to a heat lamp, **infrared** uses infrared radiation to warm the superficial tissue and create a general feeling of relaxation and pain relief. **Paraffin treatment** involves dipping a patient's involved body part (usually hands or feet) into a mixture of melted paraffin wax and mineral oil that is maintained at a temperature of approximately 135° F. The heat from the paraffin produces the relaxing and pain-reducing effects of other superficial heat treatments, and also leaves the skin feeling warm and soft, allowing for greater comfort when performing range-of-motion exercises. **Fluidotherapy** is the use of a self-contained unit filled with finely-chopped corncobs into a sawdust-type substance. The particles are heated to the desired temperature and circulated by air pressure around

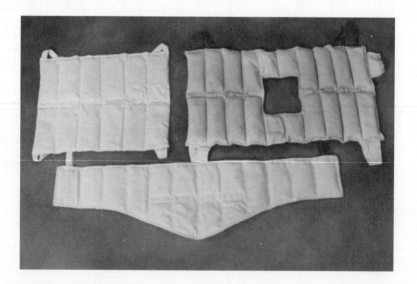

Fig. 9-9. Variety of hot packs to apply superficial heat to different body areas (Photo credit: Dewey Neild).

the involved body part. In addition to receiving the effects of heating, the patient is also able to exercise while the treatment is in progress. **Whirlpools** make use of the therapeutic effects of water by immersing the body part or entire body into a tank of water. Use of this physical agent is known as **hydrotherapy.** A variety of sizes of tanks are available, ranging from a small tank for distal extremities (Fig. 9-10) to a full-body tank known as a Hubbard Tank. In addition to its heating effects, hydrotherapy has the added advantage of assisting with wound healing.

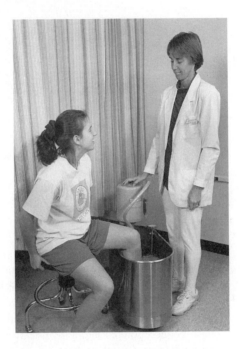

Fig. 9-10. Small whirlpool to administer hydrotherapy to a lower limb segment (Photo credit: Dewey Neild).

Deep heat modalities produce physiological effects similar to superficial heat agents, but the depth of tissues affected is deeper. Therefore, patients with deep muscle or joint dysfunctions may receive more therapeutic benefits from the application of deep heat than a superficial heating agent. Deep heat modalities include ultrasound and short wave diathermy. **Ultrasound** is the therapeutic application of high frequency sound waves that penetrate through tissue and cause an increase in the tissue temperature to promote healing and reduce pain (Fig. 9-11). Similar results are achieved with **short-wave diathermy,** although diathermy uses electromagnetic energy to produce deep therapeutic heating effects.

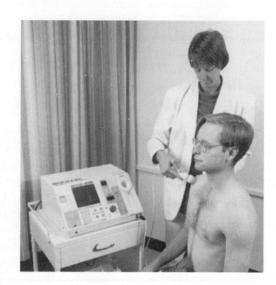

Fig. 9-11. Application of ultrasound to produce deep heat in the shoulder region (Photo credit: Dewey Neild).

In contrast to heating agents, therapeutic cold (**cryotherapy**) may be applied. Temperature differences with the application of cold agents cause a decrease in blood flow and decreased metabolism, which result in a decrease in swelling and diminished pain. Cold is the physical agent of choice in patients with acute injuries who present with clinical symptoms of swelling and/or pain (See Fig. 2-11 in Chapter 2). Cold may also be incorporated into a treatment protocol after exercises to help reduce post-exercise soreness. Cryotherapy may take the form of commercial cold packs, ice massage, cold whirlpool, or cold used in conjunction with compression.

Electrical stimulation. Physical therapists and physical therapist assistants who use physical agents as part of their treatment plans may also use electrical stimulation to achieve therapeutic results. With the use of electrical stimulation units, electrodes are placed on the skin at specified locations to stimulate nerves, muscles, and other soft tissues in attempts to reduce pain and swelling, increase strength and range of motion, and facilitate wound healing[15] (Fig. 9-12). The use of electricity to generate therapeutic benefits is not new, but the numerous electrotherapy devices on the market can make the selection of the appropriate device confusing. The therapist must have a clear understanding of the desired effects from the electrical stimulation intervention, and have knowledge of the appropriate parameters to use with regard to treatment intensity, voltage, and current type. Common physical agents used in electrotherapy are listed in Table 9-2.

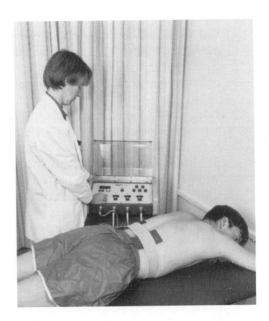

Fig. 9-12. Use of transcutaneous electrical nerve stimulation (TENS) for treatment of pain in the low back region. (Photo credit: Dewey Neild).

Other physical agents. Additional physical agents that may be used in the treatment of orthopaedic patients include: mechanical traction, hyperbaric oxygen, biofeedback, laser, and ultraviolet. These modalities achieve therapeutic benefits through mechanisms different than thermal or electrical, but may also be used to decrease a patient's pain or improve strength or motion in an attempt to maximize function.

Manual techniques

Physical therapists working with orthopaedic patients always have two tools at their ready disposal—their hands. Perhaps in no other patient population is touch so important as it is in the orthopaedic population. Whether palpating a structure during an evaluation, providing manual force for a patient to resist against when exercising, or performing a mobilization to increase range of motion, a therapist's hands are an important therapeutic instrument. A variety of manual techniques are currently being used by orthopaedic physical therapists, and many of these techniques are the subject of clinical research in order to validate and clarify their purpose and clinical efficacy.

For the purpose of this text, manual techniques will be divided into two categories: soft tissue mobilization and joint mobilization. It is beyond the scope of this text to cover specific procedures and the schools of thought behind the various techniques. The reader is again referred to the reading list at the end of this chapter for further information regarding this topic.

Soft Tissue Mobilization. Soft tissue mobilizations include a variety of "hands-on" techniques designed to improve movement and function. The techniques are designed to decrease pain or swelling and relax muscle or fascia tension in order to create proper postural alignment and optimal muscle function.

Two common forms of soft tissue mobilization are massage and myofascial release. **Massage** involves the systematic use of various manual strokes designed to produce certain physiological, mechanical, and psychological effects. To achieve relaxation, Swedish massage strokes are used to help decrease pain or swelling, relieve tension, and improve the metabolism of surrounding tissue. More vigorous massage strokes may also be used prior to physical activity to stimulate and prepare the muscles for exertion. Another specific stroke known as transverse friction massage is useful in improving the flexibility and function of soft tissues such as muscles, ligaments, and tendons.[4]

Myofascial release involves manual stretching of the layers of the body's fascia, which is connective tissue that surrounds muscle and other soft tissues in the body[10] (See Fig. 2-8 in Chapter 2). Myofascial release techniques are thought to soften and loosen restrictions in the muscles and fascia that are limiting normal movement. These techniques are unique in that the stretching force applied by the therapist depends on the response of the patient's tissues to the stretch. The therapist must be able to "feel" facial tension diminish as a stretch is applied and adjust the amount of stretch to the patient's comfort.

Joint Mobilization. In contrast to soft tissue mobilizations which focus on stretching or relaxing soft tissue, **joint mobilization** techniques are used when a patient's dysfunction is the result of joint stiffness or hypomobility (loss of motion). Based on knowledge of the anatomy of joint surfaces and the findings from joint evaluation, the therapist applies specific passive movements to a joint, either oscillatory (rapid, repeated movements) or sustained. Joint mobilization techniques are intended to reduce the pain and stiffness affecting movement and restore normal joint motion.

Therapeutic Exercise

Therapeutic exercise has been and continues to be the foundation of a rehabilitation program. This foundation is based on scientific principles and the knowledge that the human body has the ability to react and respond to physical stresses placed upon it. In particular, the muscular and cardiovascular systems are adaptable depending on the stresses and forces placed on them. When these systems are stressed with a program of progressive exercise, positive changes will occur such as improvements in strength and endurance. Likewise, the effects of abnormal stresses, such as prolonged bed rest, can lead to detrimental changes including osteoporosis and muscle atrophy.[8]

The goals of therapeutic exercise are not only to facilitate and restore normal function in an individual, but also to prevent an initial injury, educate the patient on how to prevent reoccurrence of an injury, and help maintain normal function. These goals are based on the results of the patient's evaluation and assessment of needs.

The level of sophistication of an exercise program should not be determined by the type of equipment the clinic may have. Some of the most sophisticated exercises can be performed with very inexpensive equipment. With creativity, many pieces of equipment can be adapted to incorporate many of the goals of therapeutic exercise. This section will describe a variety of therapeutic exercise techniques that may be used with a patient who has an orthopaedic dysfunction. These include exercises to improve range of motion, strength, flexibility, balance and coordination, cardiovascular endurance, and function.

Range-of-Motion Exercise. As mentioned earlier in the chapter, range-of-motion exercises can be categorized into two types: PROM and AROM. Passive range of motion may be provided manually by the therapist, or mechanically by a machine. This type of exercise might be used with (but not limited to) patients who are restricted to bed rest, who have paralysis of one or more limbs, or are in a coma. It may also be used when AROM is contraindicated. Active range of motion can be subdivided into active-assisted movement, active-free movement, and active-resisted movement. When performing **active-assisted ROM,** the patient may be assisted either manually or mechanically if the prime muscle mover is weak (Fig. 9-13A). Pendulum exercises are an example of **active-free ROM,** in which the patient does not receive any support or resistance (Fig. 9-13B). In **active-resisted exercises,** an external force resists the movement. The last category includes a variety of techniques, several of which are described in the next section.

Resisted Exercise. Resisted exercise is a form of active movement in which some form of resistance is provided.[4] The goals of a resisted exercise program are to increase muscular strength and endurance. **Muscular strength** refers to the maximal amount of tension an individual can produce in one repetition. **Muscle endurance** refers to the ability to produce and sustain tension over a prolonged period of time.[5] If the goal is to increase strength, then the program would concentrate on low repetitions using heavy resistance. If the goal is to increase endurance, then the exercise program would concentrate on using low resistance for high repetitions. The type of exercise performed depends on the types of activities to which the patient is planning to return. When designing a program, the therapist must also consider the type(s) of resisted exercise on which the patient should concentrate. Resisted exercise can be categorized into three types: isometric, isotonic, and isokinetic.[4] Definitions and examples of these types are outlined in Table 9-3. Typically, a combination of all three types of exercise is necessary to perform any type of functional activity.

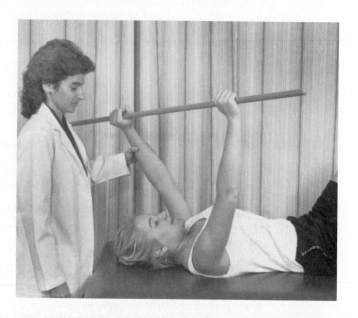

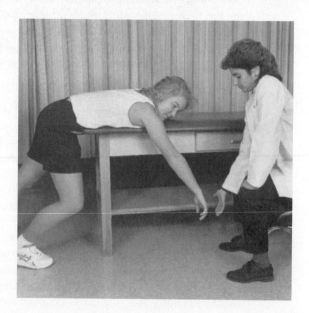

Fig. 9-13. Range-of-motion exercises are used to maintain/improve joint motion. **A.** A cane can be used to conduct simple active-assistive range-of-motion exercises for the shoulder. **B.** Pendulum exercises are effective active-free exercises and require no special equipment. (Photo credits: Dewey Neild).

Table 9-3. Classification of Resisted Exercises

Type of Exercise	Definition	Example
Isometric	Muscle contraction without visible joint movement	Pushing against a wall
Isotonic • concentric	Muscle contraction which produces or controls joint motion resulting in muscle *shortening*	Flexing elbow with dumbbell in hand (biceps brachii muscle)
• eccentric	Muscle contraction which produces or controls joint motion resulting in muscle *lengthening*	Extending elbow with dumbbell in hand (biceps brachii muscle)
Isokinetic	A concentric or eccentric muscle contraction which occurs at a constant speed	Knee extensions using an isokinetic device

In resisted exercise, resistance can be applied either manually by the therapist, or mechanically by the use of equipment. Manual resistance can be applied to isolated muscle groups (as is the case with manual muscle testing positions), or can be applied in patterns of movement using several muscle groups. An example of the latter is a technique called proprioceptive neuromuscular facilitation (PNF) described in Chapter 8. The use of manual resistance offers many advantages. The primary advantage is that it gives the therapist the ability to control the amount of resistance provided. This is particularly useful when working with patients who are in the early stages of rehabilitation where ROM may need to be limited and/or the patient is only able to tolerate mild to moderate resistance. The disadvantage is that it is very difficult to quantify the amount of resistance provided, and also difficult for another therapist to replicate the same amount of resistance on that patient.

There are many pieces of equipment that can be used when applying mechanical resistance. These can vary from an inexpensive strip of elastic tubing (Fig. 9-14A) to very costly and highly technological isokinetic equipment (Fig. 9-14B). Other common and frequently used equipment in the clinic includes free weights, (Fig. 9-14C) nautilus machines, and pulley systems.

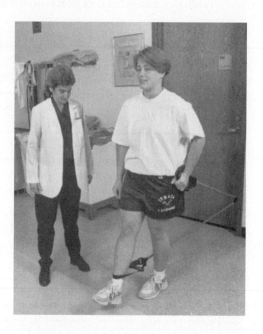

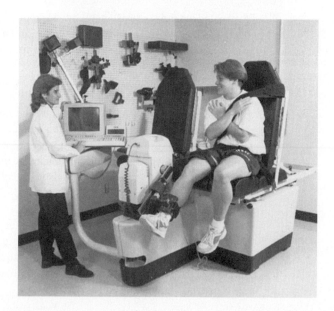

Fig. 9-14. Different methods of using mechanical resistance for exercise. **A.** Elastic tubing is inexpensive and easy to use. **B.** Isokinetic equipment is generally very expensive and sophisticated. (Photo credits: Dewey Neild).

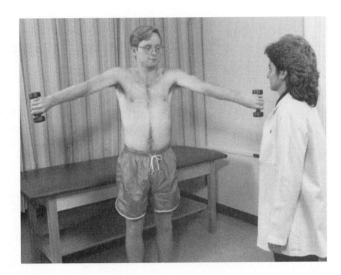

Fig. 9-14. Different methods of using mechanical resistance for exercise. **C.** Free weights are readily available to produce mechanical resistance. (Photo credits: Dewey Neild).

Flexibility Exercise. Patients recovering from a musculoskeletal injury frequently have decreased flexibility in the muscles crossing the involved joint. Conditions that may produce decreased flexibility include prolonged immobilization and tissue trauma. Many times, previous decreased flexibility may have contributed to or have been the primary cause of the injury. Therefore, flexibility is a very important component to address with the patient.

Soft tissue, such as muscle, has the ability to change length or adapt over time with stress. While there are a variety of techniques that can be used to increase flexibility, the research in this area indicates that there is no consensus on the most effective way to stretch. Further, a stretching technique that works well for one patient may be ineffective in another.

Stretching techniques can be performed passively with an external force applied either manually or mechanically. Stretching can also be performed by actively inhibiting the shortened muscle. This technique, called contract-relax, requires the shortened muscle to actively contract prior to applying a stretching force.[4]

Balance and Coordination Exercise. Proprioception is a term used to describe one's awareness of position and movement. The body is made aware of proprioception through the various receptors found in the skin and joints. These **proprioceptors** respond to stimuli such as pressure, stretch, and position. Following injury, particularly to the knee and ankle, there may be loss of proprioception, and therefore a loss in balance and/or coordination. Unfortunately, there are not many well documented tests to evaluate balance in patients with orthopaedic dysfunctions. This makes it difficult to monitor changes in balance in a rehabilitation program. However, there are numerous exercises and equipment that can be used to facilitate proper balance. One popular piece of equipment seen in the clinic is a balance board (Fig. 9-15). The patient progresses from a sitting to a standing position while shifting weight from side to side and front to back. This can also be progressed from two-legged weight shift to one-legged weight shift (balancing on one leg). The exercise can be made more challenging by having the patients close their eyes and incorporating upper extremity movement with and without weights.

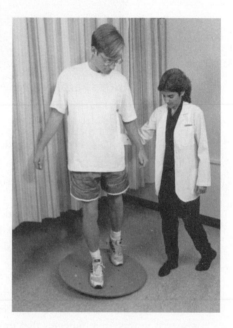

Fig. 9-15. A balance board can be used for balance exercises (Photo credit: Dewey Neild).

Cardiovascular Endurance Training. Cardiovascular or **aerobics training** refers to exercise performed over a long period of time at low intensity.[4] Aerobic exercise typically involves large muscle groups which are used in a rhythmic type of activity. There are many modes of exercise available to improve cardiovascular endurance. These include walking, running, stair climbing, cycling, cross-country skiing, and swimming. The physical therapist will choose the exercise modality that is most appropriate for the patient. For example, a patient who is recovering from a low back injury and has difficulty sitting may participate in a walking program rather than a cycling program. See Chapter 10 for a more detailed description of cardiovascular exercise.

Functional Exercises. As mentioned earlier in this chapter, the ultimate goal in physical therapy is to allow the patient to return to the prior level of function or highest level of function achievable. It is therefore imperative that exercises that mimic functional movements and activities be incorporated into the rehabilitation program. Functional movements incorporate strength, flexibility, balance and coordination. Incorporating all these factors allows patients to return to function with confidence, knowing that they performed the same or very similar exercises in the clinic.

The use of closed chain or kinetic chain exercises allows the patient to incorporate these functional movements. **Closed chain exercise** or **kinetic chain exercise** are those exercises in which movement at one joint affects the movement at other joints (e.g., a two-legged squat). **Open chain exercises** or **joint isolation exercises** are those exercises in which the end limb segment is free (e.g., biceps curl). Many of the exercises traditionally used to strengthen the lower extremity are those where the foot is off the ground. An example would be the use of isokinetic equipment for thigh strengthening. However, the lower extremity typically functions with the foot on the ground. Closed chain exercises are particularly important in the rehabilitation of the lower extremity. Therefore, exercises involving the movement of joints while the foot is on the ground facilitates proper proprioceptive feedback which mimics function (Fig. 9-16).

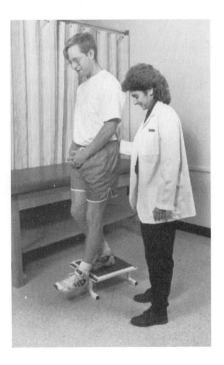

Fig. 9-16. Functional exercises, such as descending a step, are designed to mimic daily activities (Photo credit: Dewey Neild).

Home Exercise Programs

The use of therapeutic exercise in a rehabilitation program is an important and essential activity. Aside from the physical benefits derived from exercise, it also allows the patient to assume responsibility for the care of the injury and encourages active participation in the rehabilitative process. For the same reasons, home exercise programs also become a very important aspect of patient care. Treatment in the clinic two to three times per week is usually not enough time to see the desired long-lasting effects of rehabilitation, unless the patient is performing appropriate exercises, given by the physical therapist, at home. The inability of a patient to pay for physical therapy services (often due to the lack of health care insurance coverage) may also limit the number of clinic visits, making home programs even more appropriate.

Patient Education

As mentioned earlier in the chapter, communication is a critical component of the orthopaedic physical therapy experience. The therapist's depth of knowledge, effectiveness with performing and interpreting the evaluation, and the variety of treatment options available are of little value if the therapist does not share this information with patients and inform them of their role in the rehabilitation process. The patient and therapist must work together as a team, focusing on the same goals and sharing information in order to achieve optimal results.

It is the responsibility of the physical therapist and physical therapist assistant to educate the patient about exercises to perform at home, postures or positions to avoid during daily activities at work or home, and strategies to prevent dysfunctions from recurring (Fig. 9-17). In order to effectively communicate, the therapist must create a treatment atmosphere that ensures the patient's comfort and must also provide the necessary information in a clear manner that is easily understood.

It is important for the physical therapist and physical therapist assistant, when working with a patient, to treat the whole person rather than just an injured joint. Each patient comes to the therapist with a different set of values, expectations, and background. All of these factors must be considered in order to successfully and effectively treat a patient.

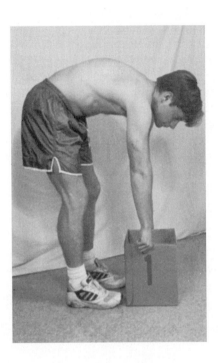

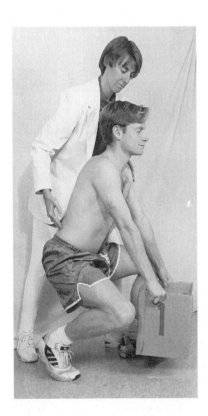

Fig. 9-17. Patient education is essential to rectify improper habits regarding body movement and posture. **A.** Improper lifting can result in a strain of lower back muscles and ligaments. **B.** Instruction in proper lifting techniques can prevent injuries to the back. (Photo credits: Dewey Neild).

CASE STUDIES

Case 1: Individual with Low Back Pain

Subjective Exam: Jack is a 36-year-old male architect who comes to the clinic with a chief complaint of left-sided lower back pain which spreads into the buttock region and occasionally down the back of his thigh. He states that the symptoms came on suddenly approximately 2 weeks ago after bending down to pick up his keys and that he had diffi-culty standing back up due to pain. He saw his physician, who recommended a course of muscle relaxants and rest. Jack states that his pain has gradually improved since onset, and he rates his pain level a "4" out of 10. The pain worsens when he lifts his 2-year-old child from the floor and with prolonged periods of sitting. He states he is able to tolerate sitting for only 10 minutes before onset of pain. Symptoms improve with walking. He has no complaints of numbness or tingling in the lower extremity. Jack sits and works at a computer approximately 5 hours/day and drives 1 hour each way to work. He reports a history of low back discomfort with prolonged sitting, but no previous history of this type of pain. Jack is not currently taking any medications. He is generally sedentary, but enjoys occasional weekend recreational activities. Jack is referred to physical therapy for evalu-ation and treatment with a diagnosis of low back pain.

Objective Exam

Observation: Posture reveals posterior pelvic tilt with slight lateral shift to the right; forward head and rounded shoulders; gait appears normal with equal weight bearing bilaterally; increased tone in spinal muscles.

ROM of lumbar spine: movement limited in all directions, with chief complaint exacer-bated with flexion movements.

Strength: Lower Extremity (LE) = Within Normal Limits (WNL); trunk muscles not tested due to pain.

Neurological Tests: reflexes 2+ (within a range of 0 to 4) and symmetrical

Special Tests: Straight Leg Raise (SLR) = Reproduces thigh pain at 40°

Goals: Primary goals of therapy were to reduce pain to enable the patient to sit for prolonged periods of time, improve ROM to functional levels, increase awareness of posture, and have patient demonstrate proper posture and body mechanics.

Treatment: Initial treatment consisted of hot packs and soft tissue massage, followed by a series of repeated lumbar extension movements while lying on stomach (prone). Jack was instructed in a gradual progression of lumbar extension exercises to be performed at home throughout the day. The patient was also instructed in proper posture during ADLs, including sleeping and sitting postures. As the pain resolved, exercises were increased to include all functional movements, flexibility exercises, and instruction in proper lifting techniques. The therapist performed a work-site analysis and made a recommendation to change the computer work station to facilitate proper alignment. Following six visits to physical therapy, Jack was discharged with a home exercise program with a recommen-dation to continue general fitness activities at the local health club.

Case 2: Individual with Fractured Radius

Subjective Exam: Alice is a 72-year-old female who sustained a fractured right radius while slipping on the ice 8 weeks ago. She was immobilized in a hand-to-mid-humeral cast with the elbow positioned in 90° of flexion, and her arm was supported in a sling for comfort. The cast was removed yesterday, and Alice states that radiographs revealed healing without any complications. She complains of stiffness and weakness throughout the upper extremity and an inability to perform daily activities such as getting dressed and preparing meals. She is right-hand dominant. Her medical history is unremarkable, her general health appears good, and she states that she remains active by walking 1 mile a day. She is referred to physical therapy for evaluation and treatment.

Objective Exam

Observation: Alice holds her upper extremity in a guarded position against her body; muscle atrophy is noted throughout the upper extremity.

AROM: Movements at the right shoulder, elbow, and wrist are limited and painful; AROM at the hand is WNL. Movements in the left upper extremity WNL.

PROM: Left upper extremity, WNL. Remaining data for right upper extremity.

> Shoulder: flexion = 0-160°
> abduction = 0-60°
> external rotation = 0-15°
> internal rotation = 0-70°
>
> Elbow: Alice is unable to extend past 60° of flexion
> Wrist: flexion = 0-45°
> extension = 0-45°

Accessory motion: Decreased glide of right glenohumeral joint.

Resisted tests: Weakness in the following muscle groups: shoulder abductors and external rotators, elbow flexors and extensors, wrist flexors and extensors.

Manual Muscle Testing (See Table 9-1 for descriptions of grades; grades are based on a scale of 0 to 5):

> Right Biceps = 4-/5   Left Biceps = 5/5
> Right Triceps = 3+/5   Left Triceps = 5/5
> No other muscles tested at this time.

Hand grip strength: Right = 15 lb, left = 25 lb

Goals: Primary goals of this patient were to restore normal movement and strength of the right upper extremity to functional levels.

Plan: Treatment for the shoulder consisted of ultrasound, followed by joint mobilizations and exercises progressing from active-assisted and active-free ROM to active-resisted. This included pendulum exercises, pulleys, and cane exercises (see Fig. 9-13).

A similar program consisting of superficial heat, joint mobilizations, and exercise was used to increase elbow and wrist ROM and strength. Proprioceptive neuromuscular facilitation (PNF) patterns (see Chapter 8) were also incorporated to facilitate functional movements at the entire upper extremity. As strength and ROM improved, simulated ADLs were added to the treatment program. This patient was seen on a regular basis for 6 weeks, and discharged with a home exercise program.

SUMMARY

This chapter has presented the role physical therapists and physical therapist assistants play in orthopaedic physical therapy. Common conditions described were overuse and traumatic injuries and surgical and medical conditions. Components of the subjective and objective exams were presented. Treatment techniques focused on physical agents, manual techniques, therapeutic exercise, home programs, and patient education. The emphasis in orthopaedic physical therapy is on assessing a patient's function and developing a treatment program that will assist the patient in returning to optimal function in the environment, whether that is on the athletic field, work site, or at home.

References

1. Bandy W: Functional rehabilitation of the athlete, Orthopaedic Clinics of North America 1(2):269-281, October 1992.

2. Barber SD, et al.: Quantitative assessment of functional limitations in normal and anterior cruciate ligament-deficient knee, Clin Orthop 255:204-214, 1990.

3. Bell BD, Hoshizak TB: Relationships of age and sex with range of motion of seventeen joint actions in humans, Can J Appl Sports Sci 6:202, 1981.

4. Cyriax J: Textbook of orthopaedic medicine, volume 1: diagnosis of soft tissue lesions, ed 8, London, 1982, Bailliere Tindall.

5. Fox E, Mathews D: The physiological basis of physical education and athletics, Philadelphia, 1981, Saunders College Publishing.

6. Gray G: Developing the lower extremity functional profile, Adrian, MI, 1994, Wynn Marketing Publications, in press.

7. Kendall FP, McCreary EK, Provance PG: Muscles testing and function, ed 4, Baltimore, 1993, Williams and Wilkins.

8. Kisner C, Colby LA: Therapeutic exercise: foundations and techniques, Philadelphia, 1990, F.A. Davis.

9. Lephart S, et al.: Relationship between selected physical characteristics and functional capacity in the anterior cruciate ligament-insufficient athlete, JOSPT 16(4):174-181, 1992.

10. Manheim CJ, Lavett DK: The myofascial release manual, Thorofare, NJ, 1989, SLACK Incorporated.

11. Michlovitz SL: Biophysical principles of heating and superficial heat agents. In Michlovitz SL: Thermal agents in rehabilitation, ed 2, Philadelphia, 1990, F.A. Davis.

12. Moffroid M, Zimny N: Causes of movement dysfunction and physical disability. In Scully RM, Barnes MR, editors: Physical therapy, Philadelphia, 1989, JB Lippincott Company.

13. Noyes FR: Objective functional testing. In Noyes FR, editor: The Noyes knee rating system, Cincinnati, 1990, Cincinnati Sports Medicine Research and Education Foundation.

14. Reed B, Zarro V: Inflammation and repair and the use of thermal agents. In Michlovitz SL, editor: Thermal agents in rehabilitation, ed 2, Philadelphia, 1990, F.A. Davis.

15. Snyder-Mackler L, Robinson AJ: Clinical electrophysiology, electrotherapy and electrophysiologic testing, Baltimore, 1989, Williams and Wilkins.

Suggested Readings

Hecox B, Mehreteab TA, Weisberg J: Physical agents: a comprehensive text for physical therapists, Norwalk, CT, 1994, Appleton and Lange. Discusses the physiological effects and application procedures for commonly used physical agents, including heat, cold, light, water, ultrasound, and electrotherapy.

Richardson J, Iglarsh ZA: Clinical orthopaedic physical therapy, Philadelphia, 1994, W.B. Saunders Company. A regional approach to evaluation and treatment of joints. Differential diagnosis and common pathologies at each joint are also discussed.

Magee D: Orthopedic physical assessment, ed 2, Philadelphia, 1992, W.B. Saunders Company. An excellent text detailing the evaluation of joints, with good descriptions of special tests.

Prentice WE: Rehabilitation techniques in sports medicine, St. Louis, 1990, Times Mirror/Mosby College. A comprehensive text discussing the implementation and profession of rehabilitation programs for sports-related injuries.

Tappan FM: Healing massage techniques: holistic, classic, and emerging methods, ed 2, Norwalk, CT, 1988, Appleton and Lange. Describes a variety of techniques and methods of massage, including the history of massage, general principles, and clinical rationale.

Evans R: Illustrated Essentials in Orthopedic Physical Assessment, St. Louis, MO, 1994, Mosby-Year Book. There are hundreds of tests for making conservative-care diagnoses of disorders of the nervous and orthopaedic systems. This manual describes them in a clearly illustrated, sequential fashion. Organization of the text is by region and specifically by presenting signs, symptoms, and indications.

Edmond S: Manipulation and Mobilization: Extremity and spinal techniques, St. Louis, MO, 1993, Mosby-Year Book.

Kennedy R: Mosby's Sports Therapy Taping Guide, St. Louis, MO, 1995, Mosby-Year Book. This practical manual offers step-by-step procedures about taping and wrapping. With over 170 illustrations and clear, descriptive instructions, this is a comprehensive manual about sports taping for the prevention and care of athletes.

Review Questions

1. What's the difference between an objective exam and a subjective one? Distinguish between the two without referring to their components!

2. Without looking at the text, how many questions can you come up with that may be helpful in a patient interview?

3. How would quantitative and qualitative measurements fit into the "SOAP" note?

4. Research some physical therapy books in your school's library to find examples of resisted tests and manual muscle testing. What, in your observation, is the main difference?

5. Try this study technique: Photocopy Table 9-2, blocking out the second column ("Physical Agents") using a folded strip of paper. Now can you fill in the applicable agents? Repeat this exercise, filling out column three instead ("Physiological Effects") or column four ("Clinical Indications"). Performing this exercise will reinforce the uses and effects of physical agents.

6. Describe the difference in purpose between exercising for muscular strength and for muscular endurance.

7. Explain why closed chain exercises are usually preferable in lower limb rehabilitation, as opposed to open chain exercises.

Chapter 10

Cardiopulmonary Physical Therapy

Ray A. Boone

*"*T*hose aspects of physical therapy commonly referred to as cardiopulmonary physical therapy are fully recognized as fundamental components of the knowledge and practice base for all entry-level physical therapists."*

EA Hillegass, PT and
HS Sadowsky, PT

KEY TERMS

angina
angioplasty
arteriosclerosis
blood gas analysis
cardiac catheterization
cardiac muscle dysfunction
cardiac pacemaker
chronic obstructive pulmonary disease (COPD)
computerized axial tomography (CAT scan)
conducting airways
congestive heart failure (CHF)
coronary artery bypass grafting (CABG)

coronary heart disease (CHD)
dyspnea
echocardiography
electrocardiogram (ECG)
embolus
exercise stress testing
expiration
heart failure
inspiration
ischemia
magnetic resonance imaging (MRI)
myocardial infarction
obstructive lung disease
pulmonary function test
respiration
restrictive lung disease
spirometer
target heart rate (THR)
training zone
ventilation

Less than thirty years ago people with cardiovascular or pulmonary disease had little hope of leading normal lives. In fact, in certain instances exercise was considered deleterious to such people. Today the physical therapist and physical therapy assistant play major roles as team members for these patient populations to enhance their function and improve the quality of their daily lives.

Physical therapists and physical therapist assistants who work with patients with cardiopulmonary disease must have a thorough understanding of the normal anatomy and physiology of these systems. Based on this knowledge, appropriate treatment programs can be developed.

GENERAL
DESCRIPTION

The Cardiovascular System

Heart. In the adult, the heart is found in the center of the chest (mediastinum) with the base located superiorly and the apex inferiorly and left of center. The major portion of the heart is made up of muscle tissue referred to as the myocardium. This muscle tissue is layered with the fibers running in multiple directions.[26]

The heart has two pairs of matched chambers. The two atria are thin-walled chambers, whereas the two ventricles have much thicker muscular walls (Fig. 10-1).[19] These chambers are separated by valves which direct the blood through the chambers in a specific pattern.

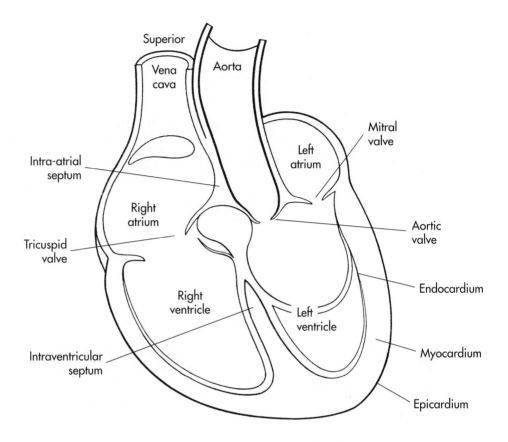

Fig. 10-1.   Schematic view of the heart, the heart chambers, and valves. (From Phillips RE, Feeney MK: The Cardiac Rhythms, ed 2, Philadelphia, 1980, WB Saunders.)

The right atrium receives venous blood from the body through the superior and inferior vena cavae. With atrial contraction (atrial systole), the blood then passes through the tricuspid valve into the right ventricle (Fig. 10-2A).[19] The left atrium receives oxygenated blood through the pulmonary veins coming from the lungs. During atrial systole, this oxygenated blood passes through the bicuspid (mitral) valve into the left ventricle (Fig. 10-2B).

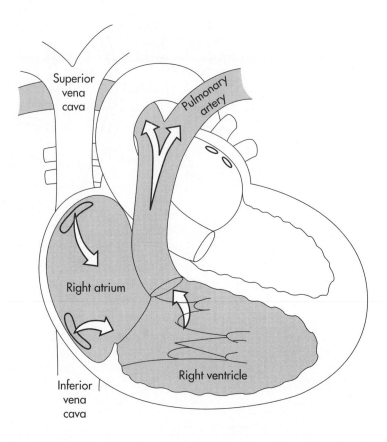

Fig. 10-2 A. Blood flow through the heart chambers. Deoxygenated blood flow from right atrium to right ventricle to the lungs through the pulmonary artery. (From Phillips RE, Feeney MK: The Cardiac Rhythms, ed 2, Philadelphia, 1980, WB Saunders.)

Once the right and left ventricles have received blood from their respective atria, ventricular contraction (ventricular systole) occurs. This results in an increase in pressure in the ventricular chambers causing the tricuspid and bicuspid valves to close tightly, preventing the blood from passing back into the atria. As ventricular contraction continues, venous blood leaves the right ventricle through the pulmonic or semilunar valve flowing into the lungs to be re-oxygenated. Oxygenated blood leaves the left ventricle through the aortic valve into the aorta to be transported to the body through the systemic circulation.

It is significant that the ventricles have thicker muscular walls than the atria. This greater muscle mass, especially in the left ventricle, must provide enough force to overcome the resistance the blood flow encounters as it moves through the peripheral arteries.[18]

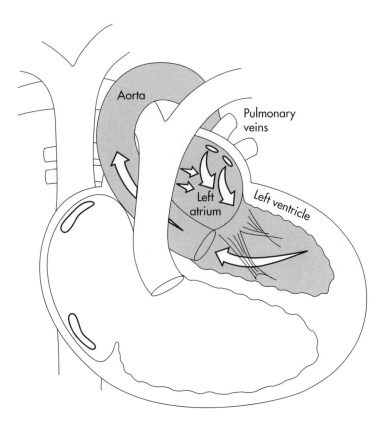

Fig. 10-2 B.   Blood flow through the heart chambers. Oxygenated blood returning to the left atrium from the lungs via the pulmonary veins, moving into the left ventricle and exiting through the aorta. (From Phillips RE, Feeney MK: The Cardiac Rhythms, ed 2, Philadelphia, 1980, WB Saunders.)

Conduction.   The myocardium contains special types of tissue which are responsible for conducting the electrical impulse that causes the myocardium to contract in a synchronized pattern. This synchronized depolarization and repolarization of the cardiac muscle results in an efficient movement of the blood through the chambers of the heart and through the coronary and peripheral vessels.

These specialized tissues are called nodal and Purkinje fibers (Fig. 10-3).[22] The sinoatrial node (SA node) initiates the impulse (sinus rhythm) and is sometimes called the pacemaker of the heart. Once the SA node initiates a signal, it travels quickly through the walls of the atria on special tracts to the atrioventricular node (AV node). The impulse also travels to the muscle fibers of the atria causing them to contract. The AV node transports the signal to the Bundle of His, which is where the Purkinje fibers start to spread out into the muscle fibers of the ventricles. For every heart beat or contraction, the depolarization signal that causes the myocardium to contract must travel through this conduction system.

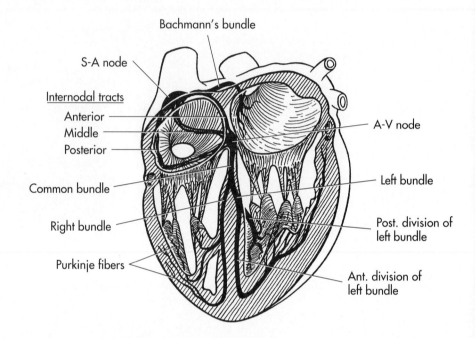

Fig. 10-3. The conduction system of the heart illustrating the location of the SA and AV nodes. (From Sanderson RG, Kurth CL: The Cardiac Patient: A Comprehensive Approach, ed 2, Philadelphia, 1983, WB Saunders.)

Both the SA and AV nodes receive autonomic nerve fibers via the sympathetic and parasympathetic systems. These nerve fibers release special neurotransmitters which influence the rate of contraction and myocardial contractility. The ability to influence the heart's rate and contractility is extremely important since this mechanism allows the central nervous system to tell the heart how to respond to increases in demand, such as those made during exercise.[18]

Coronary Arteries. The myocardium receives its blood supply from two major vessels, the right and left coronary arteries (Fig. 10-4).[16] These arteries arise from the ascending aorta, which is the major artery leaving the left ventricle carrying blood to the body (Fig. 10-1). In general, the right coronary artery carries blood to the right atrium and ventricle, whereas the left coronary artery carries blood to the left atrium and ventricle. This general pattern of blood distribution to the heart muscle varies a great deal from person to person. If something occurs which blocks a coronary vessel, it is important to determine exactly how that blockage alters the blood flow to the individual's myocardium. When a blockage occurs, the person has had a heart attack.

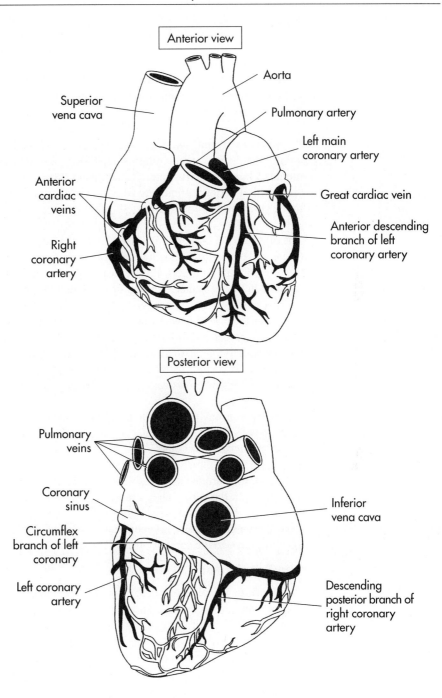

Fig. 10-4. Coronary arteries (dark shading) and veins (light shading). Note the origin of the arteries from the aorta. (From Mc Ardle WD, Katch FI, Katch VL: Exercise Physiology: Energy, Nutrition, and Human Performance, ed 3, Philadelphia, 1991, Lea and Febiger.)

Blood flow through the coronary arteries must occur when the myocardium is in a relaxed state (diastole). The pressure created during contraction (systole) is so great that blood cannot flow through the coronary vessels during this time. Therefore, if an individual can perform activities with a slow heart rate, this allows more time for blood to flow through the coronary arteries providing adequate blood and thereby oxygen to the heart muscle.[26]

Peripheral Circulation. The blood vessels which make up the peripheral circulation are arteries, veins, and capillaries. Disorders in these vessels can result in cardiopulmonary change and dysfunction, just as in other organ systems. Physical therapists work with a variety of patients who have some disability due to pathological changes in the peripheral circulation.

The arteries (the largest in diameter being the aorta) have elastic and smooth muscle tissue in their walls. This allows arteries to contract or relax. If the smooth muscle in the arterial wall contracts, this decreases the diameter of the lumen, which causes an increase in the resistance to blood flow through the artery. Arteries are often referred to as "resistance vessels." Changes in the resistance to blood flow influence how hard the heart must work to pump the blood through the body. Several factors can cause increasing resistance to blood flow in arteries. One factor is the increased activity of the sympathetic nervous system, which causes arteries to contract and decrease their lumen size. A second factor is arteriosclerosis, often referred to as "hardening of the arteries." Arteriosclerosis causes plaque to build up on the inside walls of the vessel.

The veins returning blood to the heart have much less elastic and smooth muscle tissue in their walls. The larger veins can act somewhat like a blood reservoir and are often called "capacitance vessels."

The capillaries are the smallest vessels in the peripheral circulation, and they connect the arteries to the veins. They can be so small that they will allow only one red blood cell to pass through at a time. Their walls are only one cell thick, allowing for an efficient exchange of gases (oxygen and carbon dioxide). Nutrients and waste products also pass through the capillary wall. They are often referred to as "exchange vessels."[23]

The Respiratory System

Respiration. **Respiration** is the process of exchanging oxygen and carbon dioxide between the air we breathe and the cells of the body. **Ventilation** is the process of inspiration and expiration; it results in an exchange of oxygen and carbon dioxide between the air found in the lungs and the pulmonary circulation.[6] The mechanics of inspiration and expiration depend on the muscles of respiration. The most important of these is the diaphragm. There are also muscles which have a secondary responsibility to ventilation; however, they do not generally assist the breathing process unless something interrupts the function of the primary muscles or unless disease has affected the lungs, causing an increase in the resistance to airflow.

Inspiration occurs when the muscles of respiration contract resulting in an increase in the space contained within the thoracic cavity. This expansion causes the air pressure to drop inside the lungs resulting in air moving into the lungs. **Expiration** is simply the reverse of inspiration.

If there is an increase in the need for oxygen by the cells of the body such as during exercise, the amount of air that must flow in and out of the lungs must markedly increase. When this occurs, the muscles of respiration must work much harder, and during expiration they must contract to force the air from the lungs.[23]

Conducting Airways and Lungs. Conducting airways are the passageways and tubes that transport air into or out of the lungs. The upper conducting airway includes the nose, pharynx, and larynx. This component of the air transport system cleans and humidifies the air and terminates at the beginning of the trachea. The lower conducting airway is made up of the trachea and the bronchiole system (Fig. 10-5).[23] The bronchiole system consists of tubes branching from the main bronchus out to the terminal bronchiole. It is here that the conduction system ends and the air enters into the alveolus where gas exchange takes place.

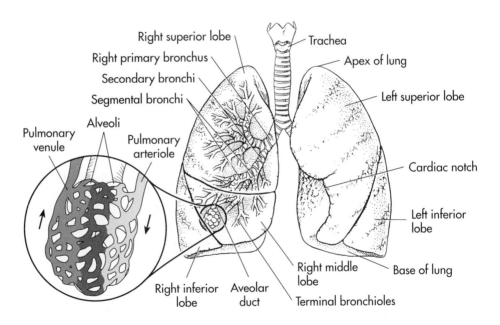

Fig. 10-5. Anterior view of the lower airway showing the bronchial tree, alveoli, and the pulmonary circulation. (From VanDeGraff KM, Fox SI: Concepts of human anatomy and physiology, ed 2, Dubuque, IA, 1988, WC Brown Publishers.)

The alveolus is surrounded by capillaries which contain the deoxygenated blood coming from the right ventricle of the heart. It is at this junction that oxygen and carbon dioxide are exchanged with the reoxygentated blood returning to the left atrium.

The lungs are compartmentalized into a system of lobes. These lobes are present due to the structure of the bronchial airway system (Fig. 10-5). A special membrane, the pleura, covers the outer surface of the lungs and the inner surface of the chest wall. The pleura is extremely important to the process of ventilation and maintaining the continuity of the lungs.[26]

Cardiovascular and Respiratory System Integration

When considering the importance of how the cardiovascular and respiratory systems interact with each other, all one has to do is realize that when disease affects one system, eventually the other system will also be affected. For example, if someone develops arteriosclerosis in the coronary vessels, this will decrease the amount of oxygen going to the heart muscle. With time, the heart muscle begins to fail and will not pump blood to the lungs and body efficiently. Eventually, this results in an increase in blood volume and pressure in the lungs, which in turn causes a decrease in lung efficiency and, finally, permanent damage.

The degree of success a physical therapist or physical therapy assistant has in establishing appropriate evaluation or treatment procedures for individuals with cardiovascular or respiratory disease depends in part on how well they understand how each system functions and interacts. The following section briefly describes common cardiovascular and lung diseases which are seen in physical therapy.

COMMON
CONDITIONS

Cardiovascular Diseases

There are two major categories of disease processes which influence the myocardium. These are ischemic conditions and cardiac muscle dysfunction.[12]

Ischemic Conditions. Ischemia occurs when there is insufficient oxygenation of tissues due to a blocked blood vessel. (If severe, an infarct, or cell death, may occur.) In cardiovascular disease, this refers to **arteriosclerosis** (hardening of the arteries) affecting the coronary vessels; it is commonly called **coronary heart disease (CHD).** **Angina** is the condition in which chest pain occurs from ischemia of the heart muscle. The clinical course or progression of this disease leads to sudden death in 20 to 25 percent of all patients or to angina.[25]

The etiology of arteriosclerosis, which can affect all vessels of the body, is not completely understood. It has been made clear, however, that the severity of the arteriosclerotic process can be influenced by many risk factors (Table 10-1).[11] Some of these factors cannot be changed, such as having a family history of CHD. However, most of these risk factors can be altered or deleted completely by changing behavior. Physical therapists and physical therapist assistants help patients with cardiac dysfunction try to alter their behavior as they progress through the rehabilitation process.

Table 10-1. Risk Factors that Promote the Development of Coronary Heart Disease*

Major Risk Factors	Minor Risk Factors
Cigarette smoking	Family history
Hypertension (High blood pressure)	Diabetes
Elevated cholesterol	Age
	Gender
	Stress
	Obesity
	Sedentary lifestyle

* Adapted from Heart and Stroke Facts, Dallas, TX, 1991, American Heart Association.

Cardiac Muscle Dysfunction. This term refers to various pathologies associated with heart failure.[12] **Heart failure** occurs when a disease process, or congenital defect, either directly or indirectly causes a decrease in the pumping capability of the heart muscle. These disease processes can occur either acutely or over time. An example of an acute change in the heart's pumping capability is the occurrence of a **myocardial infarction** (heart attack). In this case, one of the coronary arteries suddenly becomes blocked by an **embolus** (clot). When this occurs, blood flow to the heart muscle beyond the embolus stops. This results in death of that part of the heart muscle which is no longer receiving blood. If this embolus causes an interruption of blood flow to a large amount of heart muscle, death can result. Of the approximately 1.5 million myocardial infarctions in the United States per year, somewhere between 30 to 50 percent of them cause death.[25]

If an individual survives a heart attack, that person may develop other symptoms that further complicate the condition. One of the major complications following infarction is an abnormal rhythm in the sequence of heart muscle contraction (abnormal conduction). This problem makes the heart contraction very inefficient. If the left ventricle is seriously damaged from the infarct, it may not contract strongly enough to move the blood through the body appropriately. This can cause the blood to back up into the lungs or it may seriously limit function such as the heart not being able to respond to an increase in physical activity.

When the heart muscle is compromised to the point that it cannot move blood volume effectively, **congestive heart failure (CHF)** will develop. This can occur acutely or chronically. In the United States, it is estimated that over two million people suffer from CHF with 400,000 new cases occurring per year. This results in 900,000 hospitalizations each year.[12]

When CHF is present, the ventricles are not adequately pumping the appropriate amount of volume from their chambers. When the right ventricle is not contracting efficiently, blood volume backs into the venous system causing fluid to collect in the liver, abdominal cavity, and legs. If the left ventricle does not contract appropriately, then an abnormal amount of blood volume remains in the lungs, resulting in fluid collection. The right ventricle then has to work harder because it must try to push blood into the lungs against an increased resistance. This will eventually lead to compromising the function of the right ventricle (Fig. 10-2A).

A person with CHF presents many clinical problems. If fluid collects in the lungs, breathing becomes more difficult, and the blood is not oxygenated appropriately. If fluid has collected in the legs, walking becomes more difficult. With this increasing difficulty to perform, the patient would have to expend more energy to accomplish simple tasks. If this occurs, the heart would have to work harder to support simple functional activities. The physical therapist responsible for exercising a patient with these types of problems must have a thorough understanding of how these disease processes compromise function in order to develop an appropriate treatment program.

Lung Diseases

Diseases of the lung are generally classified as being obstructive or restrictive in nature. If the pathological changes in the lung cause abnormality in air flow through the bronchial tubes, then the process is defined as **obstructive lung disease.** If the pathological changes cause the volume of air in the lungs to be reduced, the process is defined as **restrictive lung disease.**[12] There still remains a great deal of controversy in how lung diseases are classified. What is most important is that the common diseases that change lung function eventually demonstrate both obstructive and restrictive characteristics.[2]

Chronic Obstructive Pulmonary Disease. Chronic obstructive pulmonary disease (COPD) is a group of disorders which produces certain specific physical symptoms. These symptoms include chronic productive cough, excessive mucus production, changes in the sound produced when air passes through the bronchial tubes, and shortness of breath **(dyspnea).** The specific disorders that can produce these changes include chronic bronchitis (inflammation of the bronchi), emphysema (trapping air in the alveoli), and peripheral airway disease (collapsing of terminal bronchioles). Other disorders that are sometimes included in this disease group include asthma (spasm-like contraction of bronchi resulting in air trapping), and cystic fibrosis (dysfunction of glands causing blockage of the bronchi).[2] The differences between these obstructive diseases include their etiology (cause), pathology (what tissues are affected and how they are changed), and management. However, all of them cause similar symptoms in varying degrees.

The signs and symptoms that develop as COPD progresses include bronchial wall abnormalities causing a decrease in lumen size and alveolar destruction. This results in trapping air in the lungs, causing them to become hyperinflated and a decrease in gas exchange in the alveoli resulting in hypoxemia (below normal oxygenation of blood). Hypoxemia occurs when the lungs cannot adequately supply oxygen to or retrieve carbon dioxide from the red blood cells as they pass by the alveoli.

As resistance to airflow increases due to the decreasing lumen size of the bronchioles, the thorax enlarges due to air trapping. This causes the respiratory muscles to work harder. With time, the effectiveness of the respiratory muscles decreases. With chronic hypoxemia, changes begin to occur in the function of the heart, blood pressure, and the thickness of the blood. All of these changes can lead to respiratory failure.[2,12]

Restrictive Lung Diseases. Restrictive lung diseases cause a decrease in the ability of the lungs to expand. This results in a decrease in the volume of air that can move into and out of the lungs. The most common cause of this disease process which effects lung tissue directly is idiopathic or unknown. Other causes include chronic inhalation of air pollutants such as coal dust, silicon or asbestos. Infections such as pneumonia, cancer of the lung, and changes in heart function (causing chronic fluid collection in the lungs) can also result in restrictive changes. Diseases or trauma to the nerve supply to the muscles of respiration or disease of the muscles themselves can also result in restriction. There are many disease groups or structural changes in the chest wall that can cause restrictive changes. Some of these affect the lung tissue itself, while others affect the chest wall or the muscles of respiration.

The signs and symptoms that develop as restrictive disease progresses include some of the same changes that are seen in COPD. These are shortness of breath and a chronic cough. However, in the case of restrictive lung disease, the cough is non-productive or does not bring mucus out of the lungs. Other changes include tachypnea or an increase in the rate of breathing resulting in a marked increase in the amount of energy expended on breathing. This increased energy cost can be so severe that it results in weight loss and the patient appears emaciated. Patients with restrictive lung disease also develop the problems associated with hypoxemia.[2,12]

EVALUATION
PRINCIPLES AND
TECHNIQUES

When the physical therapist begins the assessment of the patient with cardiopulmonary disease, data from diagnostic tests must be integrated with the patient's past medical history and other medical problems, the risk factor profile, overall history, occupation and home environment status, and family situation. The physical therapist must establish communication with the patient and family in order to determine the patient's individual needs.

Physical examination of the patient by the physical therapist specifically oriented to the cardiopulmonary system includes physical inspection of the patient, auscultation, (listening to heart and lung sounds), observation of breathing patterns, assessment of chest and muscle function, and monitoring of activity. From this process, the physical therapist will develop a plan of treatment and exercise prescription. It is significant to remember that assessment is ongoing. As the patient receives treatment and the status improves, the treatment program must respond to these improvements and change accordingly.

To be competent in developing treatment plans and managing patients with cardiopulmonary disease, a physical therapist must be capable of interpreting a variety of results from diagnostic tests and laboratory studies. Generally, the physical therapist does not participate in the technical aspect of these testing procedures. However, to understand the severity of the pathology, possible complications, and prognosis of patients with cardiopulmonary disease, it is essential that a physical therapist understand the results of many different types of testing procedures.

Cardiovascular Diagnostic Tests and Procedures

By testing the various components of the blood, several pieces of information about what has happened to a patient can be determined. For example, following a myocardial infarction, certain types of enzymes in the blood become elevated. Assessing how much increase occurs, which specific enzymes become elevated, and how long they stay elevated provides a great deal of information about the severity of the infarction. Determining the concentration of cholesterol in the blood provides information for the risk factor profile of a patient. In turn, a physical therapist can use this information to help plan the type of rehabilitation a patient will need such as special diet or exercise.

Invasive Procedures. Various pieces of equipment can be used to assess how the heart is functioning or how adequately blood is flowing through an artery. Invasive procedures used to evaluate heart function require some type of instrument to be placed in the body or injection of dye into the blood. One of the most common invasive procedures used to assess heart function is **cardiac catheterization.** The procedure requires passing a catheter (a flexible tube) into an artery in the arm or leg. The catheter is then passed along the artery reaching the heart. The catheter can then be placed in the different chambers of the heart, in the coronary arteries, in the pulmonary arteries, or in the aorta. Generally, the catheter has a special sensory device on the tip to measure pressure; thus, its use allows assessment of how much pressure is being generated in each chamber of the heart. This in turn evaluates the strength of myocardial contraction. Dye can be released directly into the coronary arteries from the catheter. A special type of imaging technique can then record how well the blood flows through the vessels and demonstrates where blockage has occurred. There are other types of invasive procedures, all of which require highly trained personnel and sophisticated equipment. These are expensive and generally involve some risk to the patient.[22]

Noninvasive Procedures. Noninvasive procedures are also used to assess heart function. Some of the more common procedures include echocardiography, electrocardiogram (ECG) monitoring, and exercise testing. **Echocardiography** is the use of high frequency ultrasound to assess the size of the heart chambers, the thickness of the chamber's walls, and the motion of the chamber walls and heart valves. Generally, the transducer (device that produces the ultrasound and records the returning echo) is placed on the chest wall. However, in some cases the transducer is placed in the esophagus to improve the accuracy of its recording and allows assessment of the posterior aspect of the heart.[22]

One of the most common and inexpensive methods of noninvasive evaluation of heart function is the **electrocardiogram (ECG).** Physical therapists who work with individuals being monitored by ECG must be able to interpret normal and abnormal ECG readings. This requires a basic understanding of the anatomy and conduction system of the heart (Fig. 10-3).

As previously discussed, the conduction system is responsible for initiating the depolarization or contraction of the heart muscle. When the conduction and muscle tissue depolarize, a change in electrical potential occurs across the individual cell membranes. This minute electrical change is detected by special electrodes placed on the skin of the anterior chest wall; this enables the "signal" to be recorded by an ECG machine (Fig. 10-6).[12]

The ECG assesses the heart's rate and rhythm (Fig. 10-7).[12] When the heart is functioning normally, it produces a consistent ECG pattern. As seen in Figure 10-7, different components of the wave form are assigned names and represent specific events of the heart cycle. For example, the P-wave represents atrial depolarization, and the QRS complex represents ventricular depolarization (contraction). If the heart does not depolarize in a normal way, or if part of the heart muscle is not functioning correctly, these would cause characteristic changes in the ECG. Other heart problems that can be assessed by ECG include heart muscle hypertrophy and the presence of myocardial infarction.[7]

Exercise stress testing is a noninvasive method of determining how the cardiovascular and pulmonary systems respond to controlled increases in activity. This technique of assessment is most frequently used to diagnose suspected or established cardiovascular disease. However, it is also valuable in other applications, such as assessing a patient's performance following coronary artery by-pass surgery or a heart valve replacement. Often the exercise stress test is used to assess someone's functional status or help prescribe limitations for occupational activities.[1]

Very often a physical therapist is involved in administering an exercise stress test. Generally, the therapist is required to have special training in the techniques of testing especially if the testing protocol requires the patient to exercise at maximum capability. At a minimum, the physical therapist must be able to interpret the data recorded during a stress test in order to establish a patient's appropriate level of exercise prescription.

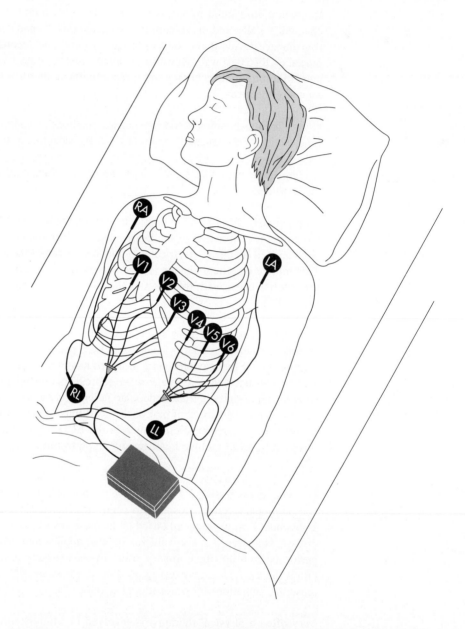

Fig. 10-6. Electrode placement for ECG monitoring. (From Hillegass EA, Sadowsky HS: Essentials of Cardiopulmonary Physical Therapy, Philadelphia, 1994, WB Saunders.)

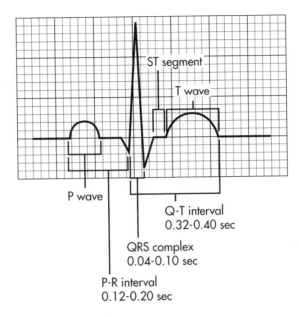

Fig. 10-7.   Normal electrocardiogram tracing during a single heart cycle. (From Hillegass EA, Sadowsky HS: Essentials of Cardiopulmonary Physical Therapy, Philadelphia, 1994, WB Saunders.)

There are several methods that can be used to administer an exercise stress test. The most common include walking on a treadmill or riding a bicycle ergometer. Generally, the actual testing procedure includes:

- continuous electrocardiogram monitoring
- heart rate monitoring (from ECG)
- blood pressure monitoring
- heart and lung sounds
- feedback from patient, reporting symptoms

In many stress test laboratories, analysis of expired gas (air) from the lungs is accomplished by having the subject breathe into a collection device. This permits the determination of the amount of oxygen the patient used during the test.[1,12]

When an exercise test is performed on a treadmill or bicycle ergometer, the exercise intensity or "protocol" which is used is very specific and has been tested in many laboratories (Table 10-2).[8] The advantage of following a protocol is that the results during the test can be compared to the results of thousands of other patients who have performed the same test. This comparison helps determine the status of the patient.

Table 10-2: Bruce Treadmill Protocol*

Stage of Exercise	Time of Each Stage (min.)	Speed of Treadmill (mph)	Grade of Treadmill
I	3	1.7	10%
II	3	2.5	12%
III	3	3.4	14%
IV	3	4.2	16%

*   Adapted from Ellestad MH, Myrvin H: Stress Testing Principles and Practice, Philadelphia, 1986, FA Davis.

Lung Diagnostic Tests and Procedures

As with cardiovascular diagnostic testing, there are invasive and noninvasive procedures that have been developed to assess lung function and the severity of pulmonary disease. Physical therapists are generally not involved in performing these assessments; however, the information that is provided must be used by physical therapists so that appropriate evaluation and treatment procedures are established.

Chest Imaging. Chest imaging is the most common non-invasive method of assessing abnormalities of the lungs. Within the last decade, new technology has enhanced the use of what are commonly called "x-rays" (radiographs). For example, **computerized axial tomography (CAT scan)** is a technique using x-rays to take pictures of small slices of the chest and lungs, then uses a computer to put these individual images into a single picture.

Magnetic Resonance Imaging. Magnetic resonance imaging (MRI) uses the same principle as the CAT scan only the energy source used to take the picture is not x-rays but magnetic waves.[17]

Even though highly technical equipment can provide a great deal of information concerning the condition of the lungs, the standard chest radiograph is often the first diagnostic test used. A physical therapist must be competent in interpreting a standard chest radiograph. Therefore, the therapist must have a thorough understanding of normal anatomy and disease processes which affect the lungs in order to assess this common diagnostic procedure.

Pulmonary Function Tests. A **pulmonary function test** is an assessment of the effectiveness of the respiratory musculature and the integrity of the airways and lung tissues. The testing procedure can help classify the lung disease pattern into obstructive or restrictive by assessing:

- lung volumes
- lung capacities
- gas distribution
- gas diffusion
- gas flow rate

Generally, in a pulmonary function test, the patient blows as hard as he/she can with the biggest possible breath into a machine called a **spirometer.** This device then measures the various volumes and airflow rates, which are then compared to a normal scale. The degree of change from normal helps assess the seriousness of the obstructive or restrictive disease.[5]

Blood Gas Analysis. Blood gas analysis involves assessing arterial blood to determine the concentration of oxygen and carbon dioxide. This helps determine how well the lungs are being ventilated or if there are any deficits in respiration. Another parameter that is assessed is the acid balance of the blood. If the lungs are having difficulty maintaining appropriate levels of oxygen and carbon dioxide, this causes the blood to generally become more acidic. In humans, the blood must be maintained at a very specific acid level. Small changes in this acid level can result in severe reactions, possibly even death.[4]

TREATMENT PRINCIPLES AND TECHNIQUES

As a team member, the physical therapist will be treating a patient in conjunction with several other personnel (e.g., doctors, nurses, nutritionists, psychologists, occupational therapists, social workers, and exercise physiologists). Each of these specialists will be applying specific management procedures. Therefore, the physical therapist must be aware of all of the treatments the patient is receiving and develop the treatment plan accordingly.

Medical Management

One of the major forms of treating heart and lung diseases is medical or pharmacological management. Each year new pharmacological agents become available to treat very specific components of the complex symptoms which develop in individuals with cardiopulmonary diseases. Generally, drugs used to treat cardiopulmonary diseases relieve or improve symptoms but do not eradicate the disease.

Understanding the effect of drugs used to treat specific heart diseases is extremely important. Many of these drugs can alter the ability of the heart to respond to exercise. For example, drugs that alter how the sympathetic nervous system influences the heart can result in a decreased heart rate and prevent the rate from increasing in response to exercise. Other drugs used to treat the heart can help control the rhythm of contraction, increase or decrease rate, and increase or decrease the strength of myocardial contraction. They can also improve coronary blood flow or help decrease the resistance to blood flow, thereby decreasing the work the heart must perform.[3]

Medical management of symptoms caused by pulmonary disease focuses primarily on promoting bronchodilation and decreasing inflammation. Drugs producing bronchodilation improve air flow through the bronchial tubes, which helps oxygen reach the alveolus and decrease the work of breathing. Antiinflammatory agents help control the results of infection or inflammation. As in the case of cardiac drugs, pulmonary drugs can have adverse effects. These affects can include alteration of heart function, gastrointestinal distress, nervousness, muscle tremor, headache, anxiety, sweating, and insomnia.[3]

Surgical Management

As in drug management, surgical management of cardiopulmonary diseases does not generally alter the disease process, but improves the quality of life by relieving symptoms. In the case of coronary heart disease, the arteriosclerotic process is not stopped, but coronary artery blood flow can be improved through surgery, and this in turn enhances heart performance.

There are two common methods used to improve coronary blood flow to the heart, angioplasty and bypass surgery. **Angioplasty,** which is the process of mechanically dilating the coronary artery, does not require surgically opening the chest. A catheter is placed through an artery in the leg and then positioned in the coronary vessel that has blockage due to an arteriosclerotic plaque. A balloon is then inflated or laser light is used to destroy the plaque.[25]

Coronary artery bypass grafting (CABG) requires surgically opening the chest wall and involves grafting a small artery or a leg vein from the aorta to a point beyond the blockage or plaque. This "bypasses" the blockage, establishing blood flow to the heart.[25]

Another major surgical intervention is heart transplant. Heart transplant is performed only when the heart has failed and all other therapies have been tried. The patient that is selected for heart transplantation is screened very carefully. The patient is generally under 60 years old, free of other diseases or infection, and is emotionally stable with strong family support. The two major problems the heart transplant patient faces is infection and rejection. If the patient overcomes these problems, survival rate at the end of one year is greater than 80 percent, and after five years is greater than 50 percent.[13,27]

Surgical intervention is also required for inserting a pacemaker. A **cardiac pacemaker** is an electronic device that produces a pulse which controls heart depolarization. In other words, it replaces the function of the SA node. This is generally done to control severe cardiac arrhythmias. Generally, the electrodes are inserted through a vein in the arm up to the heart and placed on the surface of the heart. The generator is then placed below the skin on the anterior chest wall and sutured in place. When a pacemaker is present in a patient, the physical therapist and physical therapist assistant must monitor the patient closely during exercise. Most pacemakers used today can produce variable rates in response to exercise; however, if maximum intensity exercise is done, careful monitoring must occur.[20]

Surgical management is not as frequently used for common lung diseases as it is in the management of cardiac diseases. Resection of lung disease generally applies to removal of malignant and benign tumors, fungal infections, cysts, tuberculosis, fistulas, or bronchiectasis. Pathological changes that occur from obstructive or restrictive diseases generally do not require surgery. However, when surgery on the heart or lungs is performed, the physical therapist and physical therapist assistant play a major role in pre- and post-operative care.

When the chest wall is opened, the patient generally must be placed on a machine which breathes for the individual and, in the case of heart surgery, a machine that pumps the blood. This very serious interruption of the normal function of the heart and lungs results in certain changes that will have to be managed no matter what surgical procedure is performed.[9] Box 10-1 identifies some of the problems a patient will have pre- and post-operatively that must be managed by a physical therapist.[14]

Box 10-1

Factors Influencing Recovery Following Chest Surgery*

Preoperative Factors
 Risk factor profile
 Underlying pulmonary or heart disease
 Other medical problems
Factors During Operation
 Pulmonary collapse and hypoxemia
 Direct trauma to heart or lungs
 Heart arrhythmias
 Danger of emboli (clots) in lungs
 Damage to the mucus membrane of the lungs
  Poor humidity to lungs
  Reaction of lungs to anesthesia
 Drying of pleura
Postoperative Factors
 Atelectasis (collapse of alveoli)
  Narcotics to suppress pain
  Incisional pain preventing deep breathing
  Inactivity promoting shallow breathing
 Inability to clear lung secretions due to decreased coughing
  Pain
  Weakness

* Adapted from Howell S, Hill J: Acute respiratory care in open heart surgery, Phys Ther 52 (3): 253-260, 1972.

Physical Therapy Cardiac Rehabilitation Procedures

The physical therapist is responsible for establishing an appropriate level of intensity and duration of exercise for the individual with cardiac disease. This means monitoring the patient's cardiovascular response to the exercise to ensure the patient's safety. In addition, the therapist must assess all of the medical data obtained from invasive and noninvasive testing procedures in order to select an appropriate level of activity for the patient's program.

To help the physical therapist accomplish this activity, the individual with cardiac disease is generally classified based on the severity of the condition. Table 10-3 indicates how two classification systems use functional and therapeutic terms to determine the patient's basic condition and the type of activity in which the individual might engage.[10]

Table 10-3: Functional and Therapeutic Classifications of Patients with Diseases of the Heart*

Functional Classification		Therapeutic Classification	
Level	**Description**	**Level**	**Description**
I	Patients with cardiac disease, but without resulting limitations of physical activity. Ordinary physical capacity does not cause undue fatigue, palpitation, dyspnea, or anginal pain.	A	Patients with cardiac disease whose physical activity need not be restricted in any way.
II	Patients with cardiac disease resulting in slight limitation of physical activity. Patients are comfortable at rest. Ordinary physical activity results in fatigue, palpitation, dyspnea, or anginal pain.	B	Patients with cardiac disease whose ordinary physical activity need not be restricted, but who should be advised against severe or competitive efforts.
III	Patients with cardiac disease resulting in marked limitation of physical activity. Patients are comfortable at rest. Less than ordinary physical activity causes fatigue, palpitation, dyspnea, or anginal pain.	C	Patients with cardiac disease whose ordinary physical activity should be moderately restricted and whose more strenuous efforts should be discontinued.
IV	Patients with cardiac disease resulting in inability to carry on any physical activity without discomfort. Symptoms of cardiac insufficiency or of the anginal syndrome may be present even at rest. If any physical activity is undertaken, discomfort is increased.	D	Patients with cardiac disease whose ordinary physical activity should be markedly restricted.
		E	Patients with cardiac disease who should be at complete rest or confined to bed or chair.

*   Adapted from Functional and Therapeutic Classifications of Patients with Diseases of the Heart, Dallas, TX, American Heart Association.

Other guidelines used by the physical therapist to help establish appropriate cardiac rehabilitation activities include phases of recovery. Cardiac rehabilitation is typically divided into inpatient and outpatient stages. The inpatient stage is often referred to as Phase I (acute). The outpatient stage is generally broken down into Phase II (subacute), Phase III (intensive rehabilitation), and Phase IV (ongoing rehabilitation).[12,15,25]

This classification system varies a great deal and often remains specific to a program. For instance, Phase IV is frequently combined with Phase III.

As an inpatient, the person would participate in Phase I of the cardiac rehabilitation program. Table 10-4 lists the kinds of exercises and activities of daily living (ADL) a physical therapist or physical therapist assistant would supervise or monitor.[24] The therapist or assistant must monitor the ECG, heart rate, blood pressure and other physiological parameters to ensure that the patient stays within the predetermined safety range. It is important to note that the patient is involved in educational activities, including risk factor modification, understanding the medications being taken, and discharge planning. This education program could also include flexibility exercises and learning how to take one's own pulse.

Following discharge, the individual proceeds to the outpatient phases of the cardiac rehabilitation program. These phases focus on exercises that will gradually and safely increase the individual's functional capacity. The early stages of outpatient rehabilitation (Phase II) are performed under supervision and monitored closely. Generally, patients attend outpatient cardiac rehabilitation programs that have representatives of the entire rehabilitation team (e.g., occupational therapy, physical therapy, nutrition, etc.). During Phase II, close physician management is always available. Depending on the severity of the problem, the patient will attend supervised training sessions three to four times per week for ten to twelve weeks. If recovery has continued well, the patient will have a stress test to help determine how he/she has improved or responded to the exercise program.

Progression to Phases III and IV involve more independent and aggressive activities. In order to proceed to these levels, the individual must: (1) be able to self-monitor the exercise program; (2) have no contraindications to exercise; and (3) be emotionally stable.[4] These phases include a gradual increase in exercise intensities. Periodic checkups by the professional team occur most frequently in Phase III. Once the patient has reached Phase IV, he/she should be functioning at the maximum safe capacity.

During the outpatient phases of the cardiac rehabilitation program, the exercises emphasize aerobic training which includes rhythmic activity of large muscle masses. Appropriate aerobic training involves a warm-up period, a peak period and a cool-down period. The length of time for these periods may vary depending on the status of the patient, but generally the warm-up and cool-down phases should be at least 8–10 minutes each. The peak period should last 20–60 minutes. It is during the peak period that the patient must reach and maintain a target heart rate (see below).[2,12]

Table 10-4: 7-Step Inpatient Rehabilitation Program For Myocardial Infarction*

Step	Supervised Exercises	Activities of Daily Living	Educational Activities
1.	Active and passive ROM all extremities, in bed; teach patients ankle plantar and dorsiflexion, repeat hourly when awake	Partial self-care; feed self; dangle legs on side of bed; use bedside commode	Orientation to CCU; personal emergencies; social service aid as needed
2.	Active ROM all extremities; sitting on side of bed	Sit in chair 15-30 min 2-3 times/day; complete self-care in bed	Orientation to rehabilitation team, program; smoking cessation; educational literature if requested; planning transfer from CCU
3.	Warm up exercises, stretching, calisthenics; walk 50 ft. and back at slow pace	Sit in chair; to ward class in wheelchair; walk in room	Normal cardiac anatomy and function; what happens with myocardial infarction
4.	ROM and calisthenics; walk length of hall (75 ft) and back, average pace; teach pulse counting	Out of bed as tolerated; walk to bathroom; walk to ward class; with supervision	Coronary risk factors and their control
5.	ROM and calisthenics; check pulse counting; practice walking few stairsteps; walk 300 ft bid	Walk to waiting room or telephone; walk in ward corridor	Diet; energy conservation; work simplification techniques (as needed)
6.	Continue above activities; walk down flight of stairs (return by elevator); walk 500 ft; instruct on home exercises	Tepid shower or tub bath with supervision; to occupational therapy, cardiac clinic teaching room, with supervision	Heart attack management; medications; exercise; family, community adjustments on return home
7.	Continue above activities; walk up flight of steps; walk 500 ft; continue home exercise instruction; present information regarding outpatient exercise program	Continue all previous ward activities	Discharge planning: medications, diet; return to work; community resources; educational literature; medication cards

* Adapted from Wenger NK: Rehabilitation of the Patient with Arteriosclerotic Coronary Disease. In: Hurst JN, editor: The Heart, ed 7, New York, 1990, McGraw-Hill, with permission.

A **target heart rate (THR)** is calculated as a percentage of the individual's maximum heart rate. Maximum heart rate can be accurately determined only by a maximum stress test. However, it is commonly *estimated* by subtracting one's age from 220, which is passive and non-stressful. The THR is then determined to establish a person's **"training zone"** or minimum and maximum heart rates that must be achieved to produce an aerobic training effect. The percentage of the maximum heart rate that is selected will vary based on the individual's level of fitness, symptoms, and ECG findings. If the person is a patient with cardiac disease and is very de-conditioned, then the training zone levels would be small, perhaps only 120 beats per minute or 20 to 30 beats per minute above resting levels.[12] By contrast, a training zone for a young athlete may fall between target heart rates of 60 to 85 percent of her/his maximum heart rate capacity. For this individual to produce a "training effect" or change her/his aerobic capacity, the person would have to reach a heart rate in the established "training zone." The important thing to remember is that as aerobic capacity improves, the amount of work the heart has to perform at a specific exercise intensity decreases. This in turn improves the patient's functional capacity without causing the heart to be overworked.[16]

Other factors to consider when establishing an aerobic training program besides intensity of exercise (how hard a patient works during a single exercise period) and duration of exercise (how long each exercise period should last) include mode of exercise (what the patient does such as walking, jogging, bicycle riding, etc.) and frequency of exercise (how many times a day or week the patient exercises).[1] The mode of exercise must allow for aerobic performance. This includes rhythmic contraction of large muscle groups over several minutes (20–60 minutes). Running, swimming, walking, and bicycle riding all promote this type of activity. The individual with cardiac disease, however, may not be able to sustain 20 minutes of exercise at one time; therefore, several periods of exercise throughout the day would be more appropriate. Frequency of exercise may also be determined by the patient's condition. Normally, individuals with cardiac disease in the latter phases of their program generally must perform a minimum of 20 minutes of exercise three to five times per week to promote or maintain aerobic training.[16]

The physical therapist and physical therapist assistant must continually monitor the patient during all phases of the exercise program. Appropriate monitoring includes assessing heart rate, blood pressure, and respiratory rate responses to the specific exercise intensity. This monitoring is quite important, especially in the early phases of rehabilitation since this ensures that the patient does not exercise at an unsafe level. As the patient progresses, the therapist must teach self-monitoring for safe participation in activities, moving the patient one step closer to independent activity. When the patient can function independently at maximum functional capability, the therapist's responsibilities have been met.

Physical Therapy Pulmonary Rehabilitation Procedures

As with patients who have cardiac dysfunction, the physical therapist is responsible for establishing an appropriate level of exercise programming for the individual with pulmonary disease. The intensity and duration of the program must be at an appropriate level to promote a training effort that will enhance the patient's ability to perform daily functions aerobically. Aerobic performance occurs when the active muscles receive all the oxygen they need to perform their task. To select the appropriate intensity and duration of exercise, the physical therapist must assess the results of all assessment procedures performed on the patient. From these data and the physical therapy evaluation, the appropriate exercise program can be established. It is important to remember that during aerobic exercise, the physical therapist and physical therapist assistant must monitor the cardiovascular responses to the exercise such as heart rate, blood pressure, breathing rate and depth, and the feedback from the patient on how he or she feels. In this way, excessive exercise is prevented, which could put the patient at risk.

Other components of physical therapy treatment for patients with pulmonary disease, other than exercise, include secretion removal techniques, respiratory muscle training and breathing techniques, and energy-saving techniques.

Secretion removal techniques are administered to patients who produce excessive mucus secretions, such as those seen in obstructive pulmonary disease. The technique applied to promote mucus removal is called postural drainage. The patient is placed in a certain position ("posture") to passively drain fluid from a specific portion of the lung. Percussion (or clapping), vibration, and shaking are applied by the therapist to specific areas of the chest wall overlaying specific lobes of the lung (Fig. 10-8).[21] The percussion promotes mucus to move through the bronchial tubes. Having the patient assume the Trendelenburg (inversion) position and cough immediately after the percussion or vibration procedure, also helps move the mucus out of the lower sections of the lungs.

Producing a good cough is essential for maintaining normal lung function in everyone. If the respiratory muscles are weakened or do not work properly, the efficiency of the cough mechanism is reduced. This can occur in both the obstructive and restrictive disease patterns. It also occurs in patients who have experienced trauma such as an individual with quadriplegia following spinal cord injury or patients who have had thoracic surgery.

The physical therapist can help the patient enhance coughing in three ways: by strengthening both the primary and secondary muscles of respiration; by changing the breathing pattern; and by teaching the patient how to use different devices to support the chest wall so that the expiration force generated during coughing is enhanced.[9]

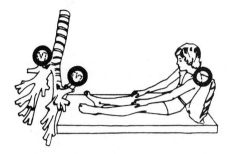

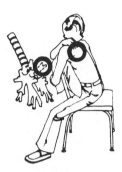

UPPER LOBES Apical Segments

Bed or drainage table flat.
Patient leans back on pillow at 30° angle against therapist.
Therapist claps with markedly cupped hand over area between clavicle and top of scapula on each side.

UPPER LOBES Posterior Segments

Bed or drainage table flat.
Patient leans over folder pillow at 30° angle.
Therapist stands behind and claps over upper back on both sides.

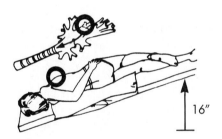

16"

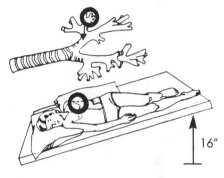

16"

RIGHT MIDDLE LOBE

Foot of table or bed elevated 16 inches.
Patient lies head down on left side and rotates 1/4 turn backward. Pillow may be placed behind from shoulder to hip. Knees should be flexed.
Therapist claps over right nipple area. In females with breast development or tenderness, use cupped hand with heel of hand under armpit and fingers extending forward beneath the breast.

LEFT UPPER LOBE Lingular Segments

Foot of table or bed elevated 16 inches.
Patient lies head down on right side and rotates 1/4 turn backward. Pillow may be placed behind from shoulder to hip. Knees should be flexed.
Therapist claps with moderately cupped hand over left nipple area. In females with breast development or tenderness, use cupped hand with heel of hand under armpit and fingers extending forward beneath the breast.

Fig. 10-8. Positions and guidelines for performing postural drainage to remove fluids from the lungs. See also Figure 2-9 A, B. (From Rothstein JM, Roy SH, Wolf SL: The Rehabilitation Specialist's Handbook, Philadelphia, 1991, FA Davis.)

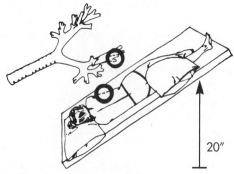

LOWER LOBES Lateral Basal Segments

Foot of table or bed elevated 20 inches.

Patient lies on abdomen, head down, then rotates 1/4 turn upward. Upper leg is flexed over a pillow for support.

Therapist claps over uppermost portion of lower ribs. (Position shown is for drainage of right lateral basal segment. To drain the left lateral basal segment, patient should lie on his right side in the same posture.)

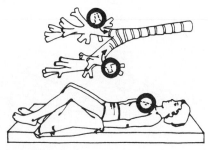

UPPER LOBES Anterior Segments

Bed or drainage table flat.

Patient lies on back with pillow under knees.

Therapist claps between clavicle and nipple on each side.

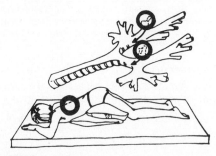

LOWER LOBES Superior Segments

Bed or table flat.

Patient lies on abdomen with two pillows under hips.

Therapist claps over middle of back at tip of scapula on either side of spine.

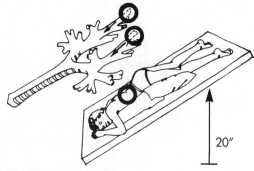

LOWER LOBES Posterior Basal Segments

Foot of table or bed elevated 20 inches.

Patient lies on abdomen, head down, with pillow under hips. Therapist claps over lower ribs close to spine on each side.

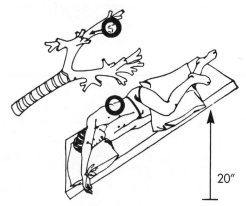

LOWER LOBES Anterior Basal Segments

Foot of table or bed elevated 20 inches.

Patient lies on side, head down, pillow under knees.

Therapist claps with slightly cupped hand over lower ribs. (Position shown is for drainage of left anterior basal segment. To drain the right anterior basal segment, patient should lie on his left side in same posture.)

Fig. 10-8. *Continued.*

Patients are taught energy-saving techniques so that they can perform their daily activities more efficiently, thereby decreasing the demand on the pulmonary system. The physical therapist assesses the activity needs for the patient in the home or work environment and then helps select assistive devices that can be used to perform certain tasks. Examples of such devices include a bath tub seat for showering in a seated position or a long shoe horn to help make putting on shoes easier. The therapist also teaches these patients how to break an activity into components so that each part of an activity is performed in stages. This is sometimes referred to as pacing.[2,9,12]

The physical therapist and physical therapist assistant engage in direct intervention during pulmonary rehabilitation. They also participate in helping modify the patient's risk factor profile, such as promoting weight management, good nutrition, smoking cessation, and a positive psychological state. They must be prepared to monitor the activities of other health care professionals and ensure that their treatment program is integrated into a comprehensive care plan. The primary goal for pulmonary rehabilitation is to help the patient achieve the highest functional level allowed by the pulmonary impairment.

The "Well" Individual

A discussion of cardiopulmonary physical therapy would not be complete without reviewing the concept of the "well" individual (individual without a diagnosis of any cardiopulmonary disease). These individuals may be candidates for fitness programs aimed at improving their functional work capacity. A physical therapist or physical therapy assistant needs to be prepared to offer guidance to this type of person. Generally, these exercise programs focus on a specific purpose for starting exercise. These may include stress reduction, weight management, improving physique and body image, alteration of cardiac risk factors, or enhancing functional capacity.[12]

The aging population represents a large group of "well" individuals who can benefit from exercise but have a tendency to be sedentary. Specific cardiopulmonary changes occur with aging. One of the most specific cardiac changes is a decrease in safe maximum heart rate. It is well established that heart rate is inversely related to age. As one grows older, heart rate declines. At the same time, the pulmonary system demonstrates a decline in both static and dynamic measurements. However, while endurance training in the elderly cannot reduce cardiac changes, it can reduce pulmonary changes.[16]

Just as an individual with cardiac or pulmonary disease needs an assessment, so does the "well" individual. This assessment should include reviewing the risk factor profile including smoking and family history. The physical therapist should evaluate the functional status of the musculoskeletal system. The performance results of an exercise stress test, body composition (percentage of body fat), strength and flexibility should also be assessed. Any preexisting conditions, such as orthopaedic abnormalities, must also be considered. An important aspect of the assessment is to determine the individual's specific interests. Does the individual like to swim, run, or ride a bicycle? Understanding this will help the person comply with the exercise routine.

Box 10-2 presents a summary of benefits gained from aerobic and strength training programs.[12] This type of information can be used to encourage a sedentary person to engage in a regular exercise program. However, appropriate assessment and monitoring must accompany any regular exercise.

Box 10-2

Benefits of Aerobic Exercise and Strength Training Programs*

Benefits of an Aerobic Exercise Program
Improvement in aerobic capacity
 Increased efficiency to extract oxygen in trained muscles
 Increase in stroke volume
 Decrease in resting heart rate
 Decrease in submaximal heart rates
Changes in body composition (loss of fat)
Decreased clotting factors in blood
Decrease in resting blood pressure in hypertensive individuals
Altered method of cholesterol transport
 Increase in high-density lipoproteins (HDLs)
 Slight decrease in low-density lipoproteins (LDLs)
Decrease in various fats produced by the body
Increase in using carbohydrates as an energy source
Improvement in psychological well-being
 Improved response to stress
 Decrease in physiologic responsiveness to stimuli
 Improved self-image
Decrease in risk for developing heart disease owing to elimination of a
 number of the risk factors

Benefits of a Strength Training Program
Increase in strength of trained muscles
Increase in utilization of anaerobic metabolism
 Improved ease in performing many activities of daily living especially
  with upper body strength training
Increase in bone mass
Increase in size, endurance, or both, of trained muscles.
Improvement of body image and self-esteem

* Adapted from Hillegass EA, Sadowski HS: Essentials of Cardiopulmonary Physical Therapy, Philadelphia, 1994, WB Saunders.

CASE STUDIES

Joe—Myocardial Infarction

Clinical History. Joe is a 60-year-old man who retired after 30 years as a high school math teacher. He had not experienced any previous symptoms of heart disease such as chest pain or shortness of breath. He had been taking medicine over the past three years for mild high blood pressure which was well controlled. His risk factor profile included:

- family history—mother and older brother died of heart disease
- smoking—between ages 16 and 40 one pack/day
- sedentary—has not engaged in any regular exercise program since age 50
- obesity—has "been carrying" an extra 30 pounds since mid-forties

One week ago, he was admitted to the emergency room following one hour of severe chest pain. The ECG demonstrated severe abnormalities indicating change in the function of the anterior-lateral part of his heart. He was rushed to the operating room where cardiac catheterization revealed major blockage in different sections of his left coronary artery. An angioplasty was performed on two areas of artery blockage, improving the blood flow through the left coronary artery by 90 percent.

Cardiac Rehabilitation. After surgery, Joe was admitted to the cardiac care unit (CCU). He was placed on medications which helped to control his heart rate, improve the strength of the heart's contractions and prevent arrhythmias. The physical therapist assessed the patient's status and, after conferring with the cardiologist and ward nurse, initiated the activities outlined in Table 10-4. The physical therapist reported the following results at the end of the exercise period:

1. Resting heart rate (bpm): 86 while lying in bed, 98 while sitting, 105 while standing, 135 while performing activities of daily living (ADL) such as brushing teeth at bedside.
2. Blood pressure: 130/90 while lying in bed, 110/80 while sitting, 110/65 while standing, 100/60 while performing ADLs.
3. ECG: no indication of change in pattern except when performing ADLs. This change demonstrated possible mild ischemia.

Following two days in the CCU, Joe was transferred to the ward. Following appropriate assessment, the physical therapist started the exercise and education programs listed in Table 10-4—for ward activities. Following the first two days of this exercise routine, the patient demonstrated appropriate physiological responses to the exercises. The physical therapist assistant assumed the responsibility for the ambulation and range-of-motion exercises. The patient was discharged following one week of hospitalization. He had an understanding that the medicine he took was to help prevent arrhythmias. He had learned how to take his own pulse and was instructed not to engage in any activities that caused his heart rate to exceed 135 beats per minute. At time of discharge, he was instructed to move his bed to the first floor of his home to avoid a flight of stairs.

Outpatient Program. Joe returned to the outpatient cardiac rehabilitation program conducted in the physical therapy department three days following discharge. He reported that he had not had any difficulty at home; however, further inquiry revealed that he did not engage in any activity other than ADLs and walking around the house.

The physical therapist initiated phase II of cardiac rehabilitation by determining how long he could walk on a treadmill at his preferred rate before reaching the target heart rate of 135 beats per minute. This was established by the cardiologist at the time of discharge as the maximum heart rate he could reach. Over the next three outpatient visits (one week), the physical therapist established the following exercise routine to be performed at home twice daily.

1. 15 minutes of warm-up and stretching
2. 20 minutes of stationary bicycle riding
3. 15 minutes of cool-down exercises

Joe remained on this exercise program for three more weeks. During that time, he came to the cardiac rehabilitation program to meet with a nutritionist and a psychologist. He then underwent an exercise stress test on a treadmill. This revealed that he could safely reach a maximum heart rate of 146 bpm before serious changes occurred in his heart function. Phase III cardiac rehabilitation was then initiated which included bicycle riding and fast walking with increasing intensity, duration, and frequency. At the end of six weeks of monitored Phase III activities, another stress test revealed that Joe could reach a safe maximum heart rate of 160 beats per minute. His resting heart rate and blood pressure were now within normal limits, he lost twenty pounds, and his diet was cholesterol free. He was no longer taking any cardiac medication. The cardiologist approved Joe's transfer into Phase IV cardiac rehabilitation with three-month checkups by the physical therapist and another stress test in one year.

Martha—COPD

Clinical History. Martha is a 58-year-old homemaker with a history of shortness of breath upon exertion. She admits to a 25-year history of smoking, but stopped five years ago. She states that she has a productive cough in the morning. Recently, she was admitted to the hospital with a temperature of 102° F and a productive cough. She was diagnosed as having severe upper respiratory tract infection. This is Martha's third such admission in the past year. Following discharge, the physician requested a full pulmonary assessment and initiation of rehabilitation in order to reduce the frequency of hospitalization.

Results of pulmonary testing revealed that her ability to forcefully expire a normal volume of air in one second was markedly decreased even though the total volume of air in her lungs remained near normal. The carbon dioxide concentration in her blood was elevated and the amount of oxygen was below normal. A chest radiograph demonstrated mild inflammation of the bronchial tubes.

The physical therapy examination of her chest revealed that her breathing pattern depended mostly on the diaphragm and very little chest wall motion. The angle her ribs form at the sternum has increased, indicating that her lower chest wall has permanently expanded beyond normal. There is evidence that her accessory muscles of respiration around the neck and shoulders contract during quiet inspiration. When Martha was placed on a treadmill and asked to walk at 3 mph with no grade, she demonstrated a further drop in the oxygen saturation of her blood, shortness of breath, and a mild wheezing.

Pulmonary Rehabilitation. Based on the assessment, Martha was diagnosed as having moderate obstructive lung disease accompanied by physical deconditioning. The primary goals for her rehabilitation program would be to achieve a daily walk/jog of 30 continuous minutes without shortness of breath, improve her functional capacity, and perform pulmonary hygiene to assist with clearing her lungs each morning.

The physical therapist instructed Martha in the appropriate postural drainage positions that she will use for 10 minutes on each side of the chest before getting out of bed in the morning. She was taught breathing exercises that will help mobilize her lower chest wall, increase the strength of her diaphragm and intercostal muscles, and improve her ability to perform a forceful cough. Martha must also learn specific diet modifications and learn how to monitor for symptoms that might occur if her blood oxygen concentration drops too severely.

Martha's exercise program includes progressive walking. The heart rate achieved when shortness of breath requires stopping will be used as the maximum heart rate. Warm-up and cool-down periods will occur before and after the continuous walking period. The duration, intensity, and frequency of the exercise program will be increased until she can achieve thirty continuous minutes of walking without shortness of breath. In conjunction with the exercise program, the physical therapist must educate the patient on how she will monitor herself safely and perform the exercise routine independently.

SUMMARY

Cardiopulmonary physical therapy has, over the past two decades, become an inherent part of the knowledge and practice base of the physical therapist. A review of the anatomy and physiology of the cardiopulmonary system reveals that a thorough understanding of how these systems function is essential to develop the skills necessary to make appropriate clinical decisions for proper assessment, management, and progression of patients with cardiopulmonary diseases. It is also essential for all physical therapists and physical therapist assistants to remember that no matter what the diagnosis, when exercise is applied as a treatment, the cardiopulmonary response to that exercise must always be monitored.

Physical therapists who work with individuals with cardiopulmonary disease must also be acutely aware of their role as team members. Whether guiding a physical therapist assistant in applying appropriate exercise intensity or discussing maximum exercise intensity levels with a cardiologist, the physical therapist must always take into account the total management program the patient with cardiopulmonary disease experiences.

References

1. American College of Sports Medicine: Guidelines for exercise testing and prescription, ed 4, Philadelphia, 1991, Lea & Febiger.

2. Brannon FJ, et al: Cardiopulmonary rehabilitation: basic theory and application, ed 2, Philadelphia, 1993, FA Davis.

3. Ciccone CD: Pharmacology in rehabilitation, Philadelphia, 1990, FA Davis.

4. Cohen S, editor: Blood gas and acid base concepts in respiratory care, New York, 1976, American Journal of Nursing Company.

5. Cohen S (editor): Pulmonary function tests in patient care, New York, 1980, American Journal of Nursing Company.

6. Dorland's medical dictionary, ed 27, Philadelphia, 1988, WB Saunders.

7. Dubin D: Rapid interpretation of EKG, ed 3, Tampa, 1974, Cover Publishing.

8. Ellestad MH, Myrvin H: Stress testing principles and practice, Philadelphia, 1986, FA Davis.

9. Frownfelter DL: Chest physical therapy and pulmonary rehabilitation, an interdisciplinary approach, ed 2, Chicago, 1987, Yearbook Medical Publishers, Inc.

10. Functional and therapeutic classifications of patients with diseases of the heart, Dallas TX, American Heart Association.

11. Heart and stroke facts, Dallas, TX, 1991, American Heart Association.

12. Hillegass EA, Sadowsky HS: Essentials of cardiopulmonary physical therapy, Philadelphia, 1994, WB Saunders.

13. Hills LD: Manual of clinical problems in cardiology, ed 3, Philadelphia, 1989, Little, Brown & Co.

14. Howell S, Hill J: Acute respiratory care in open heart surgery, Phys Ther 52(3):253-260, 1972.

15. Irwin S, Tecklin JS: Cardiopulmonary physical therapy, ed 3, St. Louis, 1995, Mosby-Year Book.

16. McArdle WD, Katch FI, Katch, FL: Exercise physiology—energy, nutrition, and human performance, ed 3, Philadelphia, 1991, Philadelphia, Lea and Febiger.

17. Minter RA: Chest imaging: an integrated approach, Baltimore, 1981, Williams & Wilkins.

18. Moore L: Clinically oriented anatomy, ed 2, Baltimore, 1985, Williams & Wilkins.

19. Phillips RE, Feeney MK: The cardiac rhythm, ed 2, Philadelphia, 1980, WB Saunders.

20. Reul GJ: Implantation of a permanent cardiac pacemaker. In Cooley DA: Techniques in cardiac surgery, ed 2, Philadelphia, 1984, WB Saunders.

21. Rothstein JM, Roy SH, Wolf SL: The rehabilitation specialist's handbook, Philadelphia, 1991, FA Davis.

22. Sanderson RG, Kurth CL: The cardiac patient: a comprehensive approach, ed 2, Philadelphia, 1983, WB Saunders.

23. Van DeGraaf KM, Fox SI:, Concepts of human anatomy and physiology, ed 2, Dubuque, IA, 1989, WC Brown Publishers.

24. Wenger NK: Rehabilitation of the patient with arteriosclerotic coronary disease. In Hearst JN, editor: The heart, ed 7, New York, 1990, McGraw-Hill.

25. Wenger NK, Hellerstein HK: Rehabilitation of the coronary patient, ed 3, New York, 1992, Churchill Livingston.

26. Williams PL, et al: Gray's anatomy, ed 36, New York, 1980, Churchville Livingston.

27. Wuff KS: Management of the cardiovascular surgery patient. In Brunner LS, Suddarth DS: Textbook of medical - surgical nursing, ed 6, Philadelphia, 1987, JB Lippincott.

Suggested Readings

Frownfelter D and Dean E: Principles and practice of cardiopulmonary physical therapy, ed 3, St. Louis, MO, 1996, Mosby-Year Book. Practical and readable, this text covers the basics of cardiopulmonary physical therapy. Throughout the text, the theme of oxygen transport is stressed. Features include key terms, review questions, and a glossary. A case studies workbook is also available.

Review Questions

1. Create a diagram that illustrates the processes of respiration and ventilation.

2. Explain why we look at the cardiovascular and respiratory systems together. Don't they have distinctly different functions?

3. Generate and label a diagram that helps you identify events associated with different components of the heart cycle.

4. Research the use of at least one of the cardiovascular or pulmonary diagnostic tools discussed in this chapter. Prepare a demonstration especially if you were able to include a visit to a treatment facility as part of your research.

5. Make up a simple description of a patient in need of cardiac rehabilitation. (A paragraph is long enough.) Then create a flow chart of the typical therapy process and the changes made as the patient progresses.

6. Repeat the steps assigned in Question 5, but this time apply it to a patient in pulmonary rehabilitation.

Chapter 11

Physical Therapy for the Older Adult

Jennifer E. Collins

> **"It is always the season for the old to learn."**
> —Aeschylus, 500 B.C.

KEY TERMS

adaptive equipment (assistive device)
dynamic balance
frail elderly
old-old
osteoarthritis
osteoporosis
presbycusis
rheumatoid arthritis
static balance
well elderly
young-old

Geriatrics, elderly, older American. What kind of individual comes to mind when these words are spoken? Is it a white-haired gentleman struggling to move a walker through long hallways? Is it a silver-haired woman swimming ten laps at the community pool?

Both of them should come to mind, as well as countless other descriptions of appearance, abilities, and challenges. In health care, professionals tend to think first of the multiple medical problems many older people have. But as physical therapists and physical therapist assistants, one may be as likely to intervene with an 85-year-old athlete as with a 70-year-old person who has had a stroke. So as the words geriatric, elderly and older person are used in this population group, consider the wide variation of possibilities for function. While keeping this individual variation in mind, the commonality is that we are all part of the aging population.

GENERAL
DESCRIPTION

Demographics

Physical therapists have provided services to individuals with conditions common to people over the age of 65 for many decades. However, only in the last decade have physical therapists and physical therapist assistants worked with older persons in such large (and growing!) numbers. Current trends in health care and life expectancy have rapidly increased the numbers of older adults requiring physical therapy services. To illustrate, in the year 1990, the population 65 years of age and older comprised 12.5% of the United States population. This represents a threefold increase since 1900. During the 1980s, this segment of the population grew at an annual growth rate of 2.2%, more than twice the rate of the total population. For those over 85 years, this growth rate was 3.5% annually.[2]

As people live longer, they tend to display more physical or medical conditions that require a physical therapist's assistance in maintaining or regaining skills necessary for maximum function in their daily activities. While each individual requiring physical therapy will benefit from specific, unique interventions, the goals for most people will include skills to independently perform such activities as bathing, cooking, dressing, and shopping. Such activities are described as activities of daily living (ADLs); more complex activities necessary for community living are called instrumental ADLs (IADLs). Tables 11-1 and 11-2 list several ADLs and IADLs, respectively, and the percent of people over 65 years of age reporting difficulties performing these activities.[24] As we can see from the percentage of people over 65 who have difficulty with transferring or walking (Table 11-1), physical therapists have an important role in improving performance of ADL.

Table 11-2 focuses specifically on the IADLs. These are skills which allow an older person to be less dependent on caregivers. For instance, shopping is a difficult skill for many people. If physical therapists provide assistive devices and provide techniques for improved balance, more individuals may be able to complete shopping trips with less assistance.

Table 11-1. Percent of Persons 65 Years of Age and Over With Reported Difficulty Performing Activities of Daily Living, by Living Arrangement, Sex, Age, and Activity: United States, 1986*

Activities of Daily Living (ADL)

| | Living Arrangement | | | |
| | Lives Alone | | Lives With Others[a] | |
Age and ADLs with difficulty	Male	Female	Male	Female
65-74 Years of Age	Percent			
Eating	1.0[c]	1.1	1.8	1.4
Toileting	4.1	2.7	2.5	2.9
Dressing	5.2	3.0	4.4	4.5
Bathing	8.6	6.3	5.6	6.6
Transferring[b]	4.2	7.4	5.8	6.4
Walking	15.8	16.1	12.1	13.1
Getting outside	7.6	8.9	5.4	7.6
75 Years and Over				
Eating	1.7[c]	1.1	1.9	4.6
Toileting	4.5[c]	7.7	4.7	11.5
Dressing	4.6[c]	7.3	6.9	13.4
Bathing	7.5	16.2	10.0	23.9
Transferring[b]	8.7	13.2	7.8	16.6
Walking	20.4	27.8	18.8	31.7
Getting outside	13.3	20.6	10.2	28.5

(Data are based on household interviews of the civilian noninstitutionalized population.)

[a] Includes spouse

[b] Getting in and out of bed or chair

[c] Persons reported as not performing an activity of daily living (ADL) are included with those reported as having difficulty with that ADL.

* From Utilization of Short Stay Hospitals, Baltimore, 1985, National Center for Health Statistics, US Department of Health and Human Services, Public Health Statistics, Series 13, No. 19, US Government Printing Office.

Table 11-2. Percent of Persons 65 Years of Age and Over With Reported Difficulty Performing Instrumental Activities of Daily Living, by Living Arrangement, Sex, Age, and Activity: United States, 1986*

Instrumental Activities of Daily Living (IADL)

| | Living Arrangement | | | |
| | Lives Alone | | Lives With Others[a] | |
Age and IADLs with difficulty	Male	Female	Male	Female
65-74 Years of Age	**Percent**			
Meal preparation	4.1	3.1	3.0	5.6
Shopping	9.9	8.8	5.0	8.6
Managing money	4.1[b]	2.0	2.4	2.6
Using telephone	2.8[b]	2.6	3.5	3.3
Light housework	3.3	3.0	3.9	6.5
Heavy housework	15.2	24.6	9.9	23.5
75 Years and Over				
Meal preparation	11.3	10.1	6.1	21.7
Shopping	15.9	23.4	12.0	30.2
Managing money	8.9	7.8	6.6	14.9
Using telephone	7.2	4.0	8.8	11.4
Light housework	13.8	11.5	8.0	21.6
Heavy housework	20.9	40.1	16.7	43.9

(Data are based on household interviews of the civilian noninstitutionalized population)

[a] Includes spouse

[b] Persons reported as not performing an instrumental activity of daily living (IADL) are included with those reported as having difficulty with that IADL.

* From Utilization of Short Stay Hospitals, Baltimore, 1985, National Center for Health Statistics, US Department of Health and Human Services, Public Health Statistics, Series 13, No. 19, US Government Printing Office.

While individual differences exist, the aging process includes changes that are common in older persons. Recent terminology developments assist professionals in differentiating groups of older adults. For instance, it has become common to refer to those people in the 65–84 age range as the **"young-old"** and those 85 years or older as the **"old-old."** Another descriptive term is the **"well elderly."** This refers to people 65 years and over who are not experiencing physical limitations or who have age-related changes that are not significant enough to affect function. The 86-year-old woman in Figure 11-1 is a good example of a person described as one of the "well elderly." While she has minor medical problems, these do not significantly affect her daily activities. In contrast, the term **"frail elderly"** is used to describe people over 65 with conditions

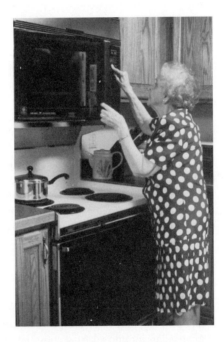

Fig. 11-1. As an example of the "well elderly," this 86-year-old woman continues to function independently at home (Photo credit: Bruce Wang).

which significantly impair their daily function.

Settings

Because the abilities and disabilities of older adults are so diverse, so are the environments in which these individuals live. Physical therapists and physical therapist assistants may work with older individuals in a wide variety of settings. People with acute medical conditions such as pneumonia, cardiovascular dysfunction, or hip fractures will be treated in hospitals. Older people with conditions such as cerebral vascular accident (stroke),

Parkinson's disease, or amputation may be seen for physical therapy in rehabilitation centers once they are medically stable. A variety of long-term care centers (skilled nursing facilities, extended care facilities, and others) provide services to older people who are not acutely ill, but who need nursing care and/or 24-hour supervision. Physical therapists and physical therapist assistants in long-term care settings provide rehabilitative services to assist people in maintaining the mobility skills they have.

Many older people with physical limitations are healthy enough to live at home and/or have family members who are able to care for them. Depending upon the medical condition of the individual and availability of appropriate transportation, older people living at home who require physical therapy may receive those services at an out-patient clinic or through a home health care agency.

Healthy older people who want to maintain their optimum physical status may attend exercise classes at senior centers or those sponsored by such groups as the Arthritis Foundation. These traditional or aquatic exercise programs may be conducted, supervised, or developed by physical therapists. The common purpose for physical therapy in all of these settings is to assist the individual in achieving functional improvement.

In each of these settings, physical therapists are educators. With valuable knowledge of the physiological aging process, physical therapists may educate patients, family members, and other professionals to assist in dispelling the myths of aging. Armed with facts, older people will be better able to exercise appropriately and maintain or regain skills. For example, the woman in Fig. 11-2 is being taught how to use her arms to more easily get up from a reclined position. The physical therapist is in an excellent position to teach the older person that strength and endurance can be increased with properly designed programs. Physical therapists can be effective advocates for older people in the areas of developing appropriate activity programs and in ensuring accessibility to all environments.

Physical therapists act as consultants to individuals and programs. For an individual, the physical therapist provides the knowledge necessary to design or acquire adaptive equipment. A piece of **adaptive equipment** (or an **assistive device**) is any device that enables an individual to accomplish a functional task with increased ease or independence. For example, a cane may assist an individual in climbing stairs safely or a bath chair may allow someone to take a bath without supervision. As a program consultant, the physical therapist makes recommendations for group activities to maintain strength and endurance. The physical therapist acts as a resource for other staff members to determine how to incorporate goals related to mobility into other components of the day program.

Aging-Related Changes

Physical therapists and physical therapist assistants must be familiar with the changes that occur in "normal" aging and with those that are pathological in nature. These changes, which vary with each individual, should be considered when conducting eval-

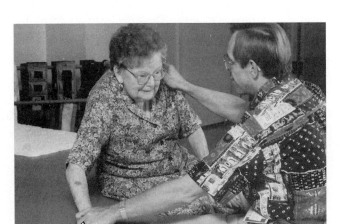

Fig. 11-2. Teaching is a major component of physical therapy. The woman in the photo is being taught how to use her arms to sit up from a reclined position (Photo credit: Bruce Wang).

uations, designing programs, and setting goals for people over 65 years of age. What is still unclear to health care practitioners is the degree to which these changes are related to reduced activity in contrast to the normal aging process. This becomes more complex as specific disease processes, which are more prevalent in the older people, are present.

Age-related changes which affect the musculoskeletal system (bones, muscles, and connective tissues) result in decreased strength, decreased flexibility, and poor posture. Decreased strength is related to hypokinesis (decreased activity or movement) and decreased muscle mass typically seen in older people. Muscle mass is reduced due to a decrease in the number of muscle fibers.[12] This reduction in fibers is related to loss of motor neurons (nerves innervating muscles) and active motor units (single motor neuron and all muscle fibers it innervates).[3]

Changes in flexibility with age are related to hypokinesis and to biological changes in connective tissue. Connective tissue tends to become less hydrated and stiffer in older persons. As older people move less and become more sedentary, the muscles are not required to lengthen and actually become shorter over time. As muscles shorten, individuals display more flexed positions which lead to postural changes.

Bone also undergoes changes with age. In studies of vertebral bodies, bone mass was shown to decrease by 35 to 40 percent between the age of 20 and 80 years.[15] This means that the bone is weaker in older people. This change may eventually advance to a condition known as osteoporosis (see Common Conditions).

The central nervous system shows a reduction in conduction velocity which is associated with age.[11] This affects the ability of the nerve to transmit impulses. This change tends to make movement responses slower in older persons and may explain the slowed gait pattern often seen in later life.

Several of the sensory systems display changes that significantly affect mobility, specifically in the ability to move safely in one's environment. The visual system is important in providing the older person accurate information regarding the environment. The lens becomes less elastic and the muscles around the lens decrease in their ability to accommodate rapidly from seeing far to near distance.[10] Visual acuity is also reduced. These changes make lighting and contrasting colors important in offering the older person more cues about objects or surfaces that might interfere with safe mobility.

Older people display a group of characteristics titled **presbycusis** ("old people's hearing"). This refers to decreased ability to perceive higher pitches and to distinguish between similar sounds.[19] Auditory acuity is also reduced. These changes are extremely important to consider when giving instructions or teaching the older person.

The tactile system is another sensory system whose changes may affect mobility. The tactile system provides important information regarding the texture and changes in the walking surface. Age-related changes reduce the amount of information the individual receives regarding the environment. If the older person does not receive accurate information regarding the surface underfoot, ambulation may become altered.

Age-related changes in the cardiovascular system are complicated by the characteristic cardiovascular diseases of old age. For example, 64 percent of people between the ages of 65 and 74 display hypertension (high blood pressure).[22] However, it appears that overall cardiac performance at rest is not altered by age in healthy people, but that cardiac response to stress does differ. This is demonstrated by a decrease in maximum cardiopulmonary function and work capacity.[18] Increased stiffness in the chest wall impacts the respiratory system which in turn, further reduces the effectiveness of cardiopulmonary function. These changes need to be considered carefully when designing exercise programs for individuals over 65 years of age.

For many years, one of the most common myths of aging was that cognitive function always significantly decreases with advanced age. In fact, people seemed to assume that dementia was inevitable. It is now known that deterioration of cognitive function characterized as dementia is related to Alzheimer's disease or some other pathological condition, not to aging itself. Reports indicate that 10 percent of the general population over 65 display dementia.[5] This increases to 20 percent in people over 85. Health professionals serving the older people should be aware of dementia and techniques for interacting with people with dementia. However, the characteristics of dementia should not be expected to be displayed universally among people over 65 or even those over 85.

Significant cognitive changes which fall in the category of normal aging are in memory and conceptualization (tasks requiring abstract thinking).[17] Specifically, there is a change in the manner in which new information is stored (encoded) in the memory. This leads to difficulty in the retrieval of newer information. However, recent studies seem to show that training in memory techniques, such as list organization, can improve recall in older persons.[16]

Finally, there are some typical psychosocial changes among people in older population groups. These vary widely based on the individual, family, environment, and presence of other changes or actual pathology. What is important for the physical therapist to remember is that psychosocial issues are extremely important to the success of any rehabilitation program. Social considerations such as adjustment to retirement, loss of lifetime roles (worker, parent, homeowner, athlete, etc.), living environment, and presence or absence of health insurance have tremendous impact on one's life. Psychologically, older persons may be required to adjust to losses of spouses, friends, and siblings. The presence of psychiatric disorders such as depression, dysthymia (disorder of mood), and anxiety is higher among homebound older people than those who are able to be out in the community.[1] The key here is that each individual will have different psychosocial characteristics to be considered.

COMMON CONDITIONS

There are many disease processes or pathological conditions more prevalent in older people which may benefit from physical therapy intervention. Individuals with the following common conditions are frequently seen by physical therapists and physical therapist assistants. (See also Parkinson's Disease and Stroke in Chapter 8.)

Arthritis

By far, the most common problem for older people is one of the joint diseases described as arthritis. In 1984, nearly 50 percent of people in the United States over 65 reported physician-diagnosed arthritis.[2] There are two primary types of arthritis. **Osteoarthritis** is characterized by degeneration of cartilage. Hands, spine, knees and hips are most commonly affected. This occurs when the cartilage deteriorates as a result of many years of use. This disease causes pain upon movement. It is important for the person with osteoarthritis to maintain at least a moderate activity level while protecting the joints.

In contrast to osteoarthritis, **rheumatoid arthritis** is a chronic inflammation of the joints of unknown etiology. While it can occur at any age, the peak incidence is between 40 and 60 years of age.[20] It is characterized by enlarged joints which are often reddened and warm to the touch. The affected joints are stiff and painful, usually more so in the morning or after extended periods of inactivity. This disease process leads to limited range of motion, joint deformity, and eventually, progressive joint destruction. Typical physical therapy goals for the person with arthritis are pain relief, increased joint movement, assistive devices, and rehabilitation when joint surgery is required.

Pain relief may be provided by heat modalities such as hot packs or paraffin baths. The physical therapist may teach the individual positioning principles for pain relief when in resting postures. Active range-of-motion exercises will be developed. Provision of assistive devices such as canes or walkers may reduce pain in the affected joints during ambulation.

If joint replacements are performed for the person with arthritis, the physical therapist will be active during the rehabilitation process. Following joint replacements, the physical therapist will provide intervention to regain muscle strength, joint motion, and activities of daily living.

Osteoporosis

Osteoporosis is another extremely common disease in older people. **Osteoporosis** is characterized by decreased mineralization of the bones. This is caused by a decreased production of new bone cells and an increased resorption of bone. Osteoporosis is more common in women than men. Other factors which predispose people to osteoporosis are being post-menopausal, family history, little physical activity, smoking, diet, and certain medications.[20] The most important problem related to osteoporosis is bone fracture. Wrist and hip fractures occur most often in the older population. The physical therapist's primary role in osteoarthritis is in prevention. This is discussed in the next section.

Hip Fracture

The combination of osteoporosis and accidental falls have made hip fracture one of the most important health care issues for older people. More than 220,000 people over the age of 65 fracture a hip each year in the United States.[24] As larger proportions of the population enter the over-65 age group, these numbers will continue to increase. Hip fracture is considered by many to be a major public health problem. A study conducted in Boston illustrates the significant impact that hip fracture has on the functional skills an elderly person may hope to regain following surgery to repair the hip. Only 33 percent of the people in that study regained their prefracture status in five basic ADLs one year after the fracture.[8] Another study showed that two months after hospital discharge, about 40 percent had regained ADLs, but only 18 percent had returned to previous levels of IADLs.[14]

Physical therapists are active in the rehabilitation of patients following hip fracture. In the hospital, transfer skills, ambulation, and use of assistive devices are taught. These skills are continued at a rehabilitation center, skilled nursing facility, or in the person's home (Fig. 11-3). As these basic skills are attained, physical therapists will then train the person to regain functional skills within the setting in which the individual will be living.

Physical therapists play an important role in the prevention of both osteoporosis and hip fractures. The most beneficial programs are directed at maintaining activity level, maintaining weight-bearing abilities, strengthening, and education regarding a safe physical

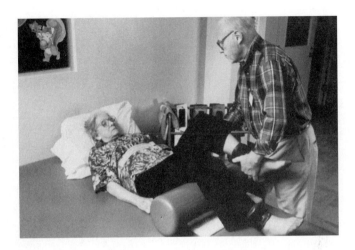

Fig. 11-3. Following instruction by the physical therapist, a volunteer provides assistance in an exercise program to regain hip and knee strength after surgery to repair a hip fracture (Photo credit: Bruce Wang).

environment. Prevention of falls requires input from the entire health care team.[9] Falls may be related to any of several medical conditions, musculoskeletal or neurological changes, side effects of medication, cognitive status, the environment, or to any combination of these factors. The health care team needs to be alert to these issues and teach the older person and family members the importance of prevention. Routine opportunities for weight bearing and walking are important as prevention strategies (Fig. 11-4).

Diabetes

Diabetes mellitus affects 10 to 20 percent of Americans over the age of 60.[13] Diabetes is a chronic disorder with effects on many body systems. It is a disease of insufficient insulin action, affecting the efficient transport of glucose into muscle, adipose, and liver cells. Glucose is not transported into these cells and accumulates in the blood. Some of the common complications of diabetes include the following: renal failure, neurological lesions (termed diabetic neuropathies), neuropathic skin ulcerations, atherosclerotic vascular disease (which makes heart attack and stroke more common in people with diabetes), and retinopathies, which may lead to blindness. Many of these complications lead to specific problems in which physical therapy may benefit the person with diabetes. For instance, foot ulcers are commonly treated by hydrotherapy, debridement, and other wound care techniques. When not responsive to treatment, foot ulcers may lead to the development of gangrene and often amputation. The rehabilitation process following an amputation requires physical therapy for stump care, prosthetic training, and gait training.

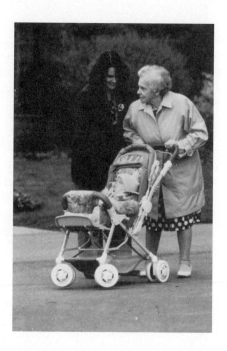

Fig. 11-4. The home care physical therapist uses another family member (child) to encourage outdoor walking as a prevention strategy (Photo credit: Bruce Wang).

For people with non-insulin dependent diabeties, management of the disease through diet and exercise is important. Physical therapists play an important role in developing exercise programs which consider the other problems of diabetes as well as other physical conditions.

EVALUATION PRINCIPLES AND TECHNIQUES

Evaluation, formal and informal, should always be the beginning of the physical therapist's intervention with an older person. The physical therapist's evaluation should be one component of a team evaluation. It is necessary for professionals from a variety of disciplines to critically observe the older person. If they all effectively share their findings, each will be able to better serve the individual.

As was pointed out earlier, older people constantly undergo a wide variety of changes after receiving services from a myriad of providers. Only if all these changes are considered and all providers are aware of the others' interventions, will treatment be of optimum benefit. However, many settings may not have every health care discipline available to its clients. In these situations, the physical therapist should be able to make observations about the individual that include not only musculoskeletal and neurological status, but also basic information regarding cognitive status, social situation, and communication abilities. Table 11-3 lists the components of a physical therapy evaluation and possible sources of data/information. Knowledge of the individual's capabilities in these areas is essential for program planning.

Table 11-3. Physical Therapy Evaluation for an Older Person

Components of Evaluation	Source of Information
Subjective Examination	Patient interview Family interview Caregiver interview
Objective Examination	Chart review Referral document Past medical history Reports from diagnostic tests
Assessment	Musculoskeletal Neuromuscular Cardiopulmonary Sensory testing Balance examination Pain examination Environmental examination ADL/Functional examination Cognitive status Psychosocial status

Evaluation should be specifically oriented to the skills and capabilities that are necessary for maximum independence. For each older person, these capabilities will differ. For example, a 70-year-old who has been inactive and sedentary since retirement at age 55 will have very different needs for rehabilitation than the 78-year-old who walks two miles every day and continues to work four hours a day as a volunteer in a recreation program. In each case, the health care team must consider the individual's function prior to the condition requiring therapy. A thorough evaluation will include information related to the person's typical daily function.

Subjective Exam

The information described above is often obtained through patient and family interview as part of the subjective examination. When interviewing the individual, the physical therapist should seek out information about how that older person views the current problem. A person's perceptions of the seriousness of the problem, the prognosis, and the course of therapy are important to consider when planning interventions and setting goals. It is also important to obtain information from the person regarding any cultur-ally based beliefs about illness, disability, and health. An older person may have very long-held beliefs that the physical therapist should consider.

Interviewing the older person will also give the physical therapist some general impres-sions of cognitive function to help determine whether a more formal examination of cognition is necessary. The individual should be able to give the physical therapist infor-mation about family support, typical activity level, occupation or former occupation, and the living environment.

Input from family members and other caregivers is important in the subjective evalua-tion. This information is very useful in determining the amount of assistance a person may need from other sources. In some circumstances, these individuals will also be able to verify information for the practitioner.

Objective Exam

The subsequent portions of the evaluation are described as objective examination (from documents) and assessment (from observation and measurement). Objective informa-tion is gained from reports, records, and patient charts. This is information such as diag-nosis, dates of hospitalization, lab reports, and other documented facts about the present illness or complaint, as well as past problems which may influence the treatment of the current problem.

Assessment of the older person (including a variety of systems and environments) will proceed much like the physical therapist's assessment of any individual, except that the physical therapist will be alert to the particular common problems of this age group. The physical therapist may adapt some examination procedures to be more appropriate to the older individual. Tasks that are requested of the individual should be explained as they relate to function. For example, the older adult may resist an activity such as creeping or kneeling on the floor. The person may be afraid of the positions or feel foolish. However, if the physical therapist explains that the activity is necessary to assess whether the person could get up from the floor if a fall occurred, the person may be more willing to cooperate.

In assessing the musculoskeletal system of the older person, the physical therapist should keep in mind the age-related changes described earlier. No studies exist to date that document what "normal" strength is in a person 65, 75, or 85 years old. The thera-pist needs to assess strength in terms of what activities the individual wants or needs to be able to perform. In other words, strength may need to be expressed in terms of func-tion. Similarly, norms for range of motion in people over 65 years have been neither established nor universally accepted. Based on the person's activity level, some reduc-tions are expected. The therapist should determine, with the older person, how much limitation of movement at the joints is acceptable. Posture can be assessed in the older adult using the same means as with other patient groups. The physical therapist should determine whether the observed posture is due to actual structural changes or whether it is a result of habit or functional issues. If the changes are not structural, education and exercise may bring significant improvement to abnormal postural findings.

The neurological examination of the older person is similar to that of any individual. There may be some slowed responses as described earlier, but it is a matter of determining what impact, if any, this has on the person's quality of life. The neurological examination should include specific sensory testing. Such testing might include two-point discrimination, proprioception, as well as visual and auditory testing performed by other members of the health care team. Sensory deficits may significantly affect functional tasks such as balance. Balance is a complex interaction of visual, perceptual, and motor skills. The physical therapist needs to assess each of these systems individually to determine which may be the cause of a balance problem.

Both static (standing still) and dynamic (while moving) balance should be examined. Techniques for examining **static balance** include observing the person standing with eyes open and eyes closed, timing of standing on one foot, and degree of postural sway. A specific balance test that can predict the likelihood of falling is the Functional Reach Test.[4] In this test, a simple measure of how far the person can reach in front of the body gives an indication of the likelihood of falls.

Dynamic balance is assessed in a number of ways. Gait is an important aspect of dynamic balance, as is functional mobility. The Tinnetti Scale tests balance and gait.[23] The Gait Abnormality Rating Scale (GARS) looks at several components of gait and relates them to balance.[25] These are just two examples of many tools available to assess balance. Gait examination should always include the use of any required assistive device and a description/consideration of the type of footwear the person uses. The type of sole or the weight of the shoe will affect the way someone ambulates. In Figure 11-5, the physical therapist is performing an initial gait examination of a gentleman approximately one month after hospital discharge following a stroke. The quadruped cane is needed at this time to assist with dynamic balance.

Information regarding balance and potential for falling is very useful to the entire interdisciplinary team working with the older person. The team will be able to develop strategies in fall prevention that range from exercise and environmental modification to teaching fall prevention skills to the older person.

Standard tests of cardiopulmonary function may be used in older persons. Older people receiving physical therapy often fatigue easily and display reduced endurance. Physical therapists assess these individuals to determine if modifications of exercise programs are necessary. Assessment of cardiopulmonary function will also help the physical therapist to determine whether goals to increase endurance are realistic and appropriate. (See also Chapter 10, "Cardiopulmonary Physical Therapy.")

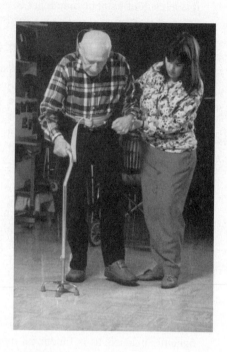

Fig. 11-5. Gait assessment using a quadruped cane following a stroke (see text; Photo credit: Bruce Wang).

Another important aspect of evaluation in the older person is pain assessment. It should be noted whether the pain is acute or chronic and whether it increases or decreases from one session to the next. In any case, it is important to assess how much discomfort the person is willing to tolerate in order to maintain independent function.

One simple means of assessing pain is on a Visual Analog Rating Scale.[21] The individual indicates the amount of pain being experienced along a 10 cm scale (see Fig. 9-2). If an objective pain index such as this is used, decreasing pain from one measurable point to another on the scale may be a very appropriate goal for an older adult. Another approach is to set a goal for a specific functional task to be performed within a tolerable level of pain.

An assessment of the environment in which the older person lives is essential. Whether the individual is in a nursing home, a relative's house, or living alone, several aspects of the environment must be considered. These include the physical layout of the living area, the access to and from the residence, and the access from the home to outside services are important. Ideally, the physical therapist should actually visit the residence rather than rely on reports from others.

The physical therapist will need to assess the access to and from the residence based on the individual's specific abilities. The following items are of importance in determining how much assistance the older person may require to be as independent in the living environment as possible:

- ground surfaces—gravel, pavement, grass, sidewalks
- curbs and curb cuts
- ramps or steps outside of home
- stairways within the home
- presence or absence of handrails
- size of door openings
- door handles, latches

This examination should be very thorough, including such items as lighting, doorways, kitchen and bathroom layout, floor coverings, furniture, and adequate space for adaptive equipment. Since there are so many items to consider, it is most efficient for the clinician to use some type of checklist for this assessment with space for individual notation.

An environmental examination is equally important whether the older person is in a private home or a long-term care facility. Long-term care facilities are obligated to ensure that residents are as free from the use of restraints as is practical. Items such as seat belts in wheelchairs, chest or hand straps in beds, and bedrails are to be used as infrequently as possible. Physical therapists in these settings are obligated to assess mobility skills and safety and make recommendations to the interdisciplinary team regarding the need, if any, for these devices. The team must first attempt to modify the physical environment to meet individual needs for safety before using restraints.

As described earlier, there are few cognitive changes that are solely a result of aging in a healthy older person. However, many of the conditions common in the elderly do have the potential for development of dementia. For this reason, the physical therapist should obtain information from other health care professionals or during the physical therapy evaluation regarding cognitive function. Cognitive abilities have great influence on how the physical therapist should provide instructions, the amount of repetition required when demonstrating, and how much practice will be required when teaching a new skill. There are standard, quick cognitive assessment tools, such as the Mini Mental Status Exam, that can easily be used by physical therapists without requiring extensive training.[7]

As in assessing all patients, it is essential that the physical therapist include psychosocial information as part of the complete evaluation of the older person. It is important to have knowledge of how the person is adjusting to the present disability. This knowledge will help the therapist determine the individual's level of motivation and whether special strategies are necessary to increase that level. An older person may see a problem such as stroke or heart attack as "the beginning of the end" and may be depressed. The therapist will benefit from knowing who the significant people are in the patient's life—spouse, family, friends.

It is also extremely important to know the setting to which the person will return, so that available social support can be determined. Social workers or business administrators are able to provide the physical therapist with pertinent details regarding each patient's specific health insurance coverage and financial status so that the impact on rehabilitation services can be considered. If only particular types of rehabilitation are covered by insurance, or if the number of paid visits is limited, the physical therapist should plan accordingly and prioritize treatment to be sure the person receives the maximum benefit from therapy.

Goals

Once subjective and objective information has been obtained, and assessments have been performed, the next step in the process of rehabilitation for the older adult is to set goals for treatment. The first consideration in establishing goals for the older person is to be sure to set goals that are meaningful for the individual and address daily function. In other words, a goal to have the person reach full or normal shoulder flexion (arm up over head to 180 degrees) may not be meaningful if the person does not have the need to reach straight up overhead. If the highest cupboards in the house require only partial flexion and the person does not put any clothing on over the head, perhaps valuable treatment time should be spent on other activities. However, if this older adult has been playing volleyball two times a week and wants to return to doing so, then full shoulder flexion is very important.

To set goals which are meaningful and functional, the older person needs to be involved throughout the process. This may require some encouragement from the professional, especially if the person believes that the role of the health care professional is to issue direction and to wait for patient compliance. Many older people feel it is not the role of the patient to determine treatment. The professional should be prepared to help the older adult be more involved in decision making regarding care.

The interdisciplinary approach mentioned throughout this chapter is also important when setting goals. The individual may have multiple medical and rehabilitative needs. The team, including the patient and family, should examine all of those needs and prioritize which should be addressed initially and which are more long term in nature.

TREATMENT PRINCIPLES AND TECHNIQUES

Physical therapy for any patient should focus on the problems identified from the evaluation; however, care for the older person requires emphasis in certain areas. These include (1) education, (2) intervention techniques with the expectation of improved function, (3) modification of accepted treatment techniques as necessary for the effects of aging, (4) recommendation of environmental modification, (5) training in the use of appropriate adaptive equipment, and (6) setting.

Education

Education of the older person should be both general and specific. General, factual information about the effects of aging on the various body systems will give the older person a good background and model from which to judge the changes which that individual may experience. This information will help the older person appreciate the importance of achieving or maintaining an active life style in order to prevent those changes that are linked to being inactive. More specific information pertaining to the particular problem the older adult is experiencing is also important. Such topics as the typical course of the disorder, expected type and length of treatment, expectations for the home program, and impact on function should be clearly outlined.

Education plays a role in motivating older adults; however, other techniques can help motivation as well. Often, older people will enjoy therapy if social interaction can be built into the process. Establishing a group of people with similar abilities for exercise may be very beneficial and fun! Designing treatment in such a way that the person is competing, either with results of the last treatment session or with peers, may also serve to increase motivation to perform.

For some individuals, motivation will not be an issue at all. These people may be very motivated, but not confident in their own abilities to carry out a program when the therapist works with another person, or when the individual performs the program at home. Such items as lists of activities, diagrams, charts with spaces to check off, or a notebook may be very valuable in assisting this type of person to take control of the routine.

Intervention

Intervention should focus on improving the individual's function. It is important to develop treatment programs which incorporate movement patterns that normally occur during the person's routine. For example, treatment for balance problems is most beneficial if it includes such activities as balance during transitional movements (up and down from chairs, in and out of bed) and on uneven surfaces. On the other hand, one-legged standing is probably not meaningful for most older persons.

Modification of Treatment Techniques

In most cases, physical therapy protocol does not need modification based solely on aging factors. Healthy older persons can increase strength, range of motion, endurance, and overall performance using traditional approaches. For example, it has been demonstrated that 86- to 96-year-old nursing home residents who underwent exercise (resistance training) programs were able to increase quadriceps strength.[6] In Figure 11-6, the woman is engaged in resistive exercise to increase strength in hip and knee musculature. Modification may be necessary, however, based on the presence of medical conditions. Cardiovascular and cardiopulmonary conditions, arthritis, and diabetes are all examples of conditions common in older individuals, for which modifications of accepted treatment protocols might be necessary. The physical therapist and physical therapist assistant working with the elderly should be alert to these and be prepared to intervene appropriately.

Medication may also require modifications of the physical therapy treatment. Some medications affect the ability to perform physical activity. Frequently, older people take multiple medications, both prescribed and over-the-counter. The physical therapist

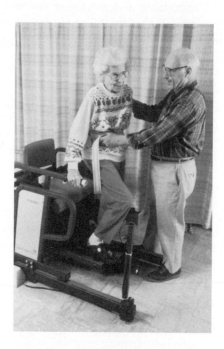

Fig. 11-6. Resistive exercises to increase strength, in this case in the hip and knee musculature, are effective in the elderly (Photo credit: Bruce Wang).

should be aware of the medications being taken by the individual, possible drug interactions, and side effects of the medication. For example, many drugs have dizziness as a side effect. If the physical therapist is working with someone on activities such as getting out of bed, getting up from the floor, or more advanced balance activities, it is essential that the therapist be alert to any signs of dizziness. If the person is taking medication that may increase dizziness, it may be necessary for the physical therapist to take increased safety precautions while performing these activities. For information related to medical conditions and medications, the physical therapist should remain in close contact with the physician and other team members.

Environmental Modification/Adaptive Equipment

While treating an older person, the physical therapist should keep the need for environmental modification and adaptive equipment in mind. Simple changes in the environment (improved lighting, removal of throw rugs, or furniture re-arrangement) may make the individual more functional in the living environment. Appropriate adaptive equipment and training in its use may enable the older person to be more independent. Training in adaptive equipment should include demonstration and repeated opportunities to practice.

Setting

A final consideration in designing treatment for the older person is the setting. In a physical therapy department, there are usually multiple pieces of equipment to achieve improved strength and mobility or to decrease pain. However, in this setting, the physical therapist may have to be creative to ensure that enhanced performance on objective tests will actually result in improvement in daily function. Physical therapy in the home setting provides the opposite challenge. There will be many opportunities in a home to improve functional skills, but it may be difficult to increase strength or endurance over long distance. The therapist must keep these advantages and limitations in mind when planning treatment programs. In Figure 11-7, parallel bars are used to assist the woman in gait training. When she is ready to return to a home environment, another device, such as a walker, may be necessary in order to increase the distance she is able to walk.

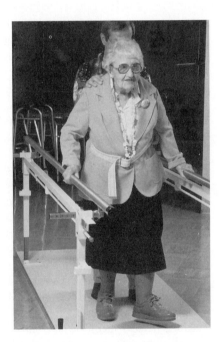

Fig. 11-7. Gait training is enhanced by using parallel bars in a clinical setting (Photo credit: Bruce Wang).

CASE STUDY

This example is provided with the intent of demonstrating the complex medical, cognitive, psychosocial, and ethical issues that face the health care practitioner who works with older people and their families.

Margaret Evans is an 81-year-old woman who has been hospitalized for seven days following a total hip replacement. She has the multiple diagnoses of rheumatoid arthritis, osteoporosis, and hypertension. She is also hearing impaired. The arthritis causes her almost constant pain in her hips, knees, and hands. The surgery was performed to relieve pain in her right hip, which was the side displaying more severe pain. Mrs. Evans lives alone in her home where she has resided for 40 years. Payment on her home mortgage was completed six years ago. Her husband is deceased, her son lives 250 miles away, and her daughter lives with her family about 10 miles away. Mrs. Evans has a limited income (Social Security) and her medical coverage is Medicare.

Mrs. Evans is considered medically ready for discharge from the hospital. She has been receiving physical therapy once a day for the following: (1) range of motion to all extremities, focusing on hip and knee musculature; (2) transfer training (moving from wheelchair to toilet, bed to standing, etc.); and (3) gait training with a walker. The physical therapist made a home visit and noted the following: (1) there are four steps into the house; (2) the bedroom Mrs. Evans uses is upstairs (13 steps); (3) there are many throw rugs on the hardwood floors; (4) the bathrooms both have tubs with showers; and (5) the laundry facilities are in the basement.

Mrs. Evans wants to go home as soon as possible. She has never been away from her home more than three days and has been very lonely for her neighbors while in the hospital. She sometimes awakes at night disoriented and confused about where she is. Her daughter, who works full time, is concerned about her mother's safety at home and is not sure whether her mother is ready to go home alone. She has also stated that she wants to be sure her mother has every opportunity for full rehabilitation and is advocating for daily physical therapy.

The team, including Mrs. Evans and her daughter, meet to discuss a discharge plan. A short-term placement is proposed. In this plan, Mrs. Evans would be discharged to a skilled nursing facility where daily physical therapy could be provided. Mrs. Evans is opposed to that move, although her daughter tries to convince her that it is a good proposal. The social worker suggests discharge to home and asks the team what other support services are necessary to ensure her success at home. The physical therapist indicates that Mrs. Evans should learn to navigate stairs safely with crutches, obtain adaptive equipment such as a bathing chair and a raised toilet seat, and modify the home environment in order to be successful at home. Physical therapy services could be provided two to three times weekly through a home health care agency. The social worker suggests that a home health aide would be appropriate to assist Mrs. Evans with personal care, housework, and laundry. These services would all be covered by Medicare as long as her physical condition causes her to be homebound.

Mrs. Evans is pleased, but her daughter is still concerned for the safety of her mother. The rehabilitation nurse suggests an emergency call button for Mrs. Evans to obtain assistance if she falls or experiences any other urgent situation. A bedroom will be set up for her on the first floor to avoid excessive stair climbing. The team agrees to the plan, and the social worker will monitor the services on a weekly basis.

SUMMARY

As we move into the twenty-first century, the proportion of our population over age 65, and especially over 85, will continue to grow. Physical therapists and physical therapist assistants will be treating older adults in every type of setting, not solely in long-term care facilities. Certainly, there will be those who select people over 65 years as a preferred population in which to specialize, but almost all therapists and assistants will have contact with patients in this age group. In order to provide quality services to the older population, physical therapists should recognize the similarities and differences between the older person and any other individual in need of rehabilitation. The physical therapist should be able to dispel the myths related to aging, yet be ready to modify interventions as needed to address documented age-related changes. The physical therapist should be able to educate the older person requiring services and all significant others regarding the course of treatment and methods for the person to enhance function. Finally, the physical therapist must be able to communicate and cooperate with the older individuals, the family, and team members to develop a meaningful and successful plan for treatment.

The author wishes to acknowledge the staff and members of The Friendly Home in Rochester, New York, for their assistance.

References

1. Bruce ML, McNamara R: Psychiatric status among the homebound elderly: an epidemiological perspective, Am Geriatr Soc 40:561-6, 1992.

2. Chartbook on Health Data on Older Americans, Baltimore, 1993, National Center for Health Statistics, US Department of Health and Human Services, Public Health Service, Series 3, No. 29, US Government Printing Office, Baltimore, 1993.

3. Doherty TJ, et al: Effects of motor unit losses on strength in older men and woman, Appl Phys 74 (2):868-881, 1993.

4. Duncan P, et al: Clinical measure of balance, Geron 45(6):M 192-7, 1990.

5. Evans DA, et al: Prevalence of Alzheimer's Disease in a community population of older persons, JAMA 262:2551-6, 1989.

6. Fitarone MA, et al: High intensity strength training on nonagenerians: effects on skeletal muscle, JAMA 263:3029-34, 1990.

7. Folstein MF, et al: Mini mental state: a practical method for grading the cognitive state of patients for the clinician, J Psych Res 12:189-98, 1975.

8. Jette AM, et al: Functional recovery after hip fracture, Arch Phys Med Rehab 68:735-40, 1987.

9. Kalchthaler J, Bascon R, and Quintos V: Falls in the institutionalized elderly, J Am Geriatr Soc 26:424, 1978.

10. Lewis CB: Aging: the health care challenge, Philadelphia, 1990, F.A. Davis.

11. Lewis C, Bottomly J: Geriatrics physical therapy, Norwalk, CT, 1991, Appleton and Lange.

12. Lexell J, Taylor CC, and Sjostrom L: What is the cause of the aging atrophy?, J Neur Sci 84:275-94, 1988.

13. Lipson LG: Diabetes in the Elderly: Diagnosis, pathogenesis, and therapy, Am J Med 80(suppl LA):10-21, 1986

14. Magaziner J, et al: Predictors of functional recovery one year following hospital discharge for hip fracture: a prospective study, J Geron 45(3):M101-107, 1990.

15. Mosekilde L: Normal age-related changes in bone mass, structure, and strength-consequences of the remodeling process, Dan Med Bull 40(1):65-83, March, 1993.

16. Norris MP, West RL: Activity memory and aging: the role of motor retrieval and strategic processing, Psych Aging 8(1):81-6, 1993.

17. Salthouse TA: Age related changes in basic cognitive processes. In Storundt M, VandeBos G, editors: The adult years: continuity and change, Washington, D.C., 1989, American Psychiatric Association, Inc.

18. Schneider EL, Rowe JW editors: Handbook of the biology of aging, New York, 1990, Academic Press.

19. Schaknecht HF: Pathology of the ear, Philadelphia, 1993, Lea and Febiger.

20. Schumacher HR: Primer on the rheumatic diseases, Atlanta, 1988, The Arthritis Foundation.

21. Huskisson SJ, EC: Graphic representation of pain, Pain 2:175-184, 1976.

22. Subcommittee on Definition and Prevalence of the 1984 Joint National Committee: Hypertension prevalence and the status of awareness, treatment, and control in the United States, Hypertension 7:457-68, 1985

23. Tinnetti M: Performance oriented assessment of mobility problems in elderly patients, J Am Ger Soc 34 (2):119-26, 1986.

24. Utilization of short stay hospitals, Baltimore, 1985, National Center for Health Statistics, US Department of Health and Human Services, Public Health Service, Series 13, No. 19, US Government Printing Office.

25. Wolffson L, et al: Gait assessment in the elderly: a gait abnormality rating scale and its relation to falls, J Geron 45(1):M12-19, 1990.

Suggested Readings

Goldstein TS: Geriatric orthopaedics, Gaithersburg, Md, 1991, Aspen Publishers. Musculoskeletal problems of older individuals are addressed in depth. Clinical management of these problems is described with an emphasis on exercise suggestions. The information is organized according to the involved joint.

Guccione AA: Geriatric physical therapy, St. Louis, 1994, Mosby-Year Book. This textbook, aimed at the entry level physical therapy student, provides information necessary to guide the professional in treatment of the older patient. It addresses assessment methods and modification of these for the people in the older age range. Common problems such as posture, falls, pain management, and wound care are examined. In addition, special population groups within the aging category are included.

Lorig K, Fries JF: The arthritis helpbook, Reading, Massachusetts, 1990, Addison-Wesley Publishing Co. Inc. The authors define and describe arthritis. However, the focus is on exercise and self-help hints. An inexpensive resource for people with arthritis.

May BJ: Home health and rehabilitation, Philadelphia, PA, 1993, F.A. Davis Co. While not written specifically for rehabilitation of older people, this book is a good source for understanding the framework of home health care. Since more patients are receiving health care in their own homes, this information is useful in developing an awareness for this aspect of the continuum of care available to aging individuals.

Schneider EL, Rowe J: Handbook of the biology of aging, New York, 1990, Academic Press, Inc. This textbook takes a scientific look at the biomedical aspects of aging. It reviews human aging research in many areas, including: cellular aging, physiology of aging, disorders in aging, and exercise in older individuals. Information is at a sophisticated level. Chapters include extensive references.

Review Questions

1. If accessible, visit both a long-term care center and an elder-care day treatment center and observe how many kinds of adaptive equipment you can see being used.

2. Explain why it is sometimes difficult for health care practitioners to determine what kinds of health changes may be due to either (a) the normal aging process, (b) reduced activity, and (c) a specific disease process. Do a little research in order to come up with at least two specific examples.

3. Challenge yourself to describe a hypothetical case in which an elderly person comes to a physical therapy clinic to be treated for conditions resulting from either arthritis, osteoporosis, hip fracture, or diabetes. Exchange "cases" with a fellow student and write about the special considerations when the patient is an older person.

4. Mr. Jamison comes to you for physical therapy that is related, he says, to his arthritis, but when you try to determine what in particular he is here for, he is very vague, only pointing out all the joints in which he "has pain off and on." Where might you look to find more specifics on his immediate needs?

5. Write two brief case scenarios that illustrate very different reasons why a treatment modification would be necessary due to an age-related consideration.

Chapter 12

Selected Topics

Michael A. Pagliarulo

> "The complexity of patient problems and the technological advances in health care, in general, have expanded the scope of practice, knowledge, and skill in the profession beyond the imagination of even twenty years ago."
>
> Colleen Kigin, PT, 1989

KEY TERMS

Acquired Immunodeficiency Syndrome (AIDS)
aquatic physical therapy
Bad Ragaz method
biological dressings
cancer
first-degree burns
full-thickness burns
functional capacity assessment
Halliwick method
heterografts
homografts
job site analysis
job task analysis
partial-thickness burns
postural examination
second-degree burns
survivor
third-degree burns

tolerances
Watsu
weighted capabilities
work-conditioning programs
work-hardening programs

The purpose of this final chapter is to provide brief and general descriptions of medical conditions or areas of practice which do not conveniently fall into one of the chapters in the practice section of this text. That is, certain conditions or practice areas are neither age related (e.g., pediatric physical therapy) nor system related (e.g., neurological physical therapy). Topics presented here are by no means exhaustive, inclusive, or comprehensive in detail. The reader is referred to other sources for detailed descriptions and intervention techniques. These topics were selected to demonstrate the diversity of physical therapy practice and highlight areas which have developed recently.

AIDS

Description

As the incidence of individuals with the **Acquired Immunodeficiency Syndrome (AIDS)** has grown, so has the population of patients with AIDS who receive physical therapy. These individuals develop neuromusculoskeletal involvement which requires physical therapy to maintain or enhance function or, at the very least, limit regression.

Although AIDS is a common medical diagnosis, it is rendered when no other cause for decreased immunity can be identified.[4] The individual with this diagnosis must test positively for the human immunodeficiency virus (HIV) and have an opportunistic infection or malignancy. The medical management focuses on chemotherapy. Physical management is dependent upon the dysfunction.

Physical Therapy Intervention

Musculoskeletal Involvement. The primary symptom regarding muscle dysfunction is that of fatigue. While strength may test generally well, it is the endurance characteristic of muscle performance that is limited.[4] Physical therapy intervention should focus on body mechanics and activities of daily living to produce efficient movement.

Pain Syndromes. Pain is frequently associated with the disease. The etiology varies from the side effects of chemotherapy to trigger points from the muscle atrophy.[4] Treatment includes physical agents (e.g., TENS—see Chapter 9) and manual therapies (e.g., myofascial release techniques).

Neurological Involvement. The involvement of the nervous system is extensive, to the point that some authors believe this disease should be considered a neuromuscular degenerative disorder.[5] The brain, spinal cord, and peripheral nerves are all involved. This results in weakness, incoordination of movement, dementia, and psychiatric disorders. Physical therapy intervention would therefore, include a broad spectrum of activities such as developmental activities, exercise, and assistive devices to maintain the highest level of function possible.

Cardiopulmonary Involvement. While cardiac muscle may become involved, the most common opportunistic infection is *pneumocystis carinii pneumonia.*[4] This results in decreased pulmonary function and further deterioration of endurance. Physical therapy intervention would follow the principles and techniques for patients with pulmonary diseases as described in Chapter 10.

HIV-Infected Child

Unfortunately, the incidence of AIDS in the pediatric age group is increasing. This is a result of maternal infection during pregnancy. As with the adult population, these individuals present with neuromuscular and pulmonary disorders. Normal motor and sensory function must be correlated to the chronological age of the child. These individuals, including newborns, present with developmental delays, delayed or absent postural reactions, pathological reflexes, and spasticity.[9] Other complications include difficulty in feeding and respiratory functions. Physical therapy intervention incorporates those principles and techniques described in Chapters 7 and 10 to address the neuromuscular and pulmonary dysfunctions, respectively.

Ethics

Are physical therapists and physical therapist assistants ethically obligated to treat an individual who is infected with HIV or has AIDS? This is a difficult question to answer. The Code of Ethics and Standards of Ethical Conduct for the Physical Therapist Assistant, which bind all members of the American Physical Therapy Association (APTA), address the issues of rights and dignity of all individuals and health needs of the public (see Boxes 5-1, 5-2). Moreover, the House of Delegates of the APTA adopted a position in 1989 to address this issue (Box 12-1).[14] While the title is generic to all infectious diseases, it certainly applies to individuals who are HIV positive or who have AIDS.

Box 12-1

Position on Infectious Diseases*

Physical therapy practitioners have an obligation to provide quality, nonjudgmental care in accordance with their knowledge and expertise to all persons who need it, regardless of the nature of the health problem. When providing care to individuals, the Association advocates that members be guided in their actions by guidelines developed by the Centers for Disease Control and Prevention (CDC) and regulations set by the Occupational Safety and Health Administration (OSHA).

* Position on infectious diseases, HOD 06-89-39-84, Alexandria, VA, 1989, American Physical Therapy Association.

The APTA policy indicates that "physical therapy practitioners" are obligated to treat individuals with infectious diseases. It stipulates, however, that this should be done in accordance with certain federal guidelines which include appropriate testing and universal precautions procedures. Sim and Purtillo agree and provide several arguments to support this from the perspectives of ethics, morality, and responsibility.[17]

AQUATIC
PHYSICAL
THERAPY

Description

The origins of the use of water for therapeutic use date back to the ancient Greeks and Romans using therapeutic baths.[20] "Pool therapy" developed in the 1920s in the United States as part of the therapeutic program for children with poliomyelitis (see Fig. 1-4). President Franklin D. Roosevelt was instrumental in promoting this type of therapy, as he frequently visited the resort in Warm Springs, Georgia, to receive "pool therapy" for his poliomyelitis. As polio declined with the introduction of vaccines, so did the therapeutic use of pools. More recently, however, aquatic therapy has been shown to be beneficial for a variety of orthopaedic and neurological dysfunctions. It has been distinguished from hydrotherapy and, in 1992, became a section in the APTA, Aquatic Physical Therapy Section.

The founding documents of this new Section offer a comprehensive description of this therapy (Box 12-2).[1] The description indicates that this form of therapy is effective on a variety of conditions, but also for the well individual. It is not merely a method to improve a swimming stroke, although stroke techniques may be employed. Finally, the description indicates that this is a specific skill and requires the expertise and supervision of a physical therapist.

Box 12-2

Description of Aquatic Therapy*

Aquatic Physical Therapy includes, but is not limited to, the rehabilitation, prevention, and overall wellness of a wide patient population. These patients, ranging from infants to the elderly, can benefit from safe and effective physical therapy intervention in the aquatic environment, addressing neurologic, orthopaedic, and other conditions. Aquatic physical therapy employs unique protocols but may also include swimming strokes in conjunction with specific treatment techniques. Aquatic Physical Therapy must be supervised and/or performed by a licensed physical therapist. Although various kinds of aquatic environments are utilized to perform these specific treatment techniques, Aquatic Physical Therapy is not a modality, but a procedure requiring specific skill and training to implement the aquatic techniques correctly.

* APTA Aquatic Physical Therapy Section Statement of Purposes, Rationale, and Goals, 1992, Alexandria, VA, American Physical Therapy Association.

Benefits

There are both physiological and psychological benefits to aquatic physical therapy.[8] The physiological benefits include an increase in blood supply to muscles, muscle metabolism, and respiratory rate and a decrease in blood pressure. These result when the individual exercises in water which is 92-98°F. Psychological benefits include the socialization process which accompanies group sessions in a pool. The satisfaction of success provides a boost to one's morale.

Precautions

Certain contraindications and precautions must be considered before and during any aquatic therapy session.[8] Contraindications would preclude a session for the safety of the individual (Box 12-3). Precautions focus attention on the activities of the individual. The person receiving therapy must be supervised closely to avoid fatigue and overstress of the joints and to maintain a safe position in the water.

Box 12-3

Contraindications of Aquatic Therapy*

- Fever
- Cardiac failure
- Urinary tract infections
- Open wounds

- Infectious diseases
- Contagious skin rashes
- Excessive fear of water

* Adapted from Haralson KM: Therapeutic pool programs, Clin Manage in Phys Ther 5(2):10-13, 1985.

Treatment Principles and Techniques

The beneficial effects of aquatic therapy are largely dependent on fundamental principles of physics. These include the buoyancy, viscosity, and hydrostatic pressure of the water. Creative exercises can be designed to take advantages of these effects and customize a program for a specific goal.

In addition to general exercises and manual techniques performed in the water, highly specific techniques have also been developed.[12] In the **Bad Ragaz method,** the therapist uses proprioceptive neuromuscular facilitation techniques while the patient is suspended by rings in the water environment (see Chapter 8 for a description of proprioceptive neuromuscular facilitation). The **Halliwick method** uses a preswim stroke instruction and musculoskeletal rehabilitation. **Watsu** is the application of Shiatsu in the water for relaxation. One or more of these techniques can be used effectively to improve function and performance.

BURN CARE

Caring for individuals with burns is intensive, exhaustive, and yet rewarding. Maximal functional recovery is critically dependent on early and continued physical therapy intervention.[6] Fortunately, survival rates for individuals who have been severely burned are increasing as a result of improved medical and physical management techniques. This section will address the impact of a burn on the body and how it is managed.

Pathophysiology

Classification of Burns. Burns were traditionally classified as *first, second,* or *third degree.* More recently, *partial* and *full thickness* have been used to more accurately describe the depth of the burn.[18] Overlap exists, therefore first and second are considered **partial-thickness burns** (layer of dermis is still intact). First- and second-degree burns are usually easily distinguished by the skin reactions: A **first-degree burn** results in a sunburn and a **second-degree burn** results in a blister. A **third-degree,** or **full-thickness burn,** is one that includes all the dermis.

Types. Burns have also been classified by the nature of the causative agent: thermal, electrical, or chemical.[18] It is easy to imagine the tissue destruction caused by high temperature; however, electrical and chemical burns generally cause far more internal damage than is obvious. Death may occur if vital organs are affected by the electrical current or chemical agent (through ingestion).

Percent of Area Affected. It is important to determine the percent of body area burned so that proper medical management, particularly fluid balance, can be administered. Two methods have been used. The traditional one is the Rule of Nines, whereby a body chart is used to mark the areas burned. The chart presents the body surface areas in multiples of nines. For instance, the arm (anterior and posterior surfaces) represents 9 percent; each surface of the legs (anterior and posterior) represents 9 percent; the face is 4.5 percent, etc. This method does not accurately present the proportionate body surface areas of children; therefore, a second method, the Lund-Browder chart, was developed.[18] It provides a percent breakdown of body surface area for six age categories between birth to adult. It is more accurate and can be used reliably to determine fluid intake.

Impact on Body. Burns cause destructive processes throughout several areas of the body.[18] The burned parts of the vascular system result in edema (swelling) in the affected area. Ulcers may develop in the gastrointestinal tract from stress. Fluid replacement therapy may tax the cardiopulmonary and renal systems to the point of failure. Infections can easily occur when the body's protective layer of skin is destroyed.

Treatment Principles

Medical. Immediately following a severe burn, the patient must be medically stabilized. This requires a closely monitored program of fluid therapy to replace lost fluids, maintain proper nutrition, and prevent overhydration. The unprotected area must be covered to prevent infections. This is done by a variety of methods including topical creams, closed sterile dressings, and **biological dressings.** The last category includes **homo-**

grafts (healthy skin taken from an unburned area of the patient) and **heterografts** (skin taken from other animals or artificially constructed).[18]

Psychological. Burns have dramatic impact on the mind as well as the body. Severe pain produces anxiety, withdrawal, and regression.[18] Children particularly need reassurance while family members of children need support.

Physical Therapy. A team approach to burn care is necessary; therefore, the physical therapist will continually consult with other team members to coordinate and adjust the treatment program. Physical therapy intervention begins with a thorough evaluation. Current and pre-injury physical status must be determined to initiate a treatment program. The major concerns which affect physical therapy are loss of joint mobility, decreased strength and endurance, pain, skin care, and psychosocial adjustments.[6] Treatment plans involve several activities and include positioning and splinting, exercise, and patient and family education. Proper positioning and splinting are critical to restore maximal function. Guidelines for certain resting positions have been established to prevent common deformities.[18] Exercise includes both passive and active techniques. Both are useful to maintain joint mobility while the latter is important for strength and endurance. Patient and family education is important to maintain an ongoing program and address the psychosocial impact of the burn. With multiple daily treatment sessions, the physical therapist plays a pivotal role in establishing family trust, cooperation, and program adherence.

CANCER

Description

Cancer includes a variety of diseases, all of which are characterized by uncontrolled growth and spread of abnormal cells.[13] It affects all age groups; however, the incidence is highest among adults in their mid-life or later. Survival rates depend upon the definition used. The traditional definition of a **"survivor"** or one who has been "cured", is an individual who was diagnosed with cancer and experienced a five-year or greater remission period. The National Coalition for Cancer Survivorship defines a survivor as "anyone who's received a cancer diagnosis, whether treatment is being received or has been completed."[13] According to the first definition, the survival rate is just over 50 percent. The second definition was established to be inclusive of all individuals who have or had cancer and by doing so, provides a strong advocacy group for them.

Survival rates, using the traditional definition, increase significantly with early detection. Box 12-4 indicates how the rate is lower as the disease progresses through four defined stages.[15] In some cases, cancer can be prevented such as those resulting from cigarette smoking, alcohol abuse, and sun exposure.

Box 12-4

Stages of Cancer*

Stage I: Limited to local site; resectable. Survival rate: 70% to 90%.

Stage II: Invaded organ or adjacent tissue; regional; resectable, but complete removal uncertain. Survival rate: 50%.

Stage III: Extension of Stage II with invasion into lymphatics; not resectable. Survival rate: 20% to 25%.

Stage IV: Metastatic spread beyond local site. Survival rate: 5% or less.

*   Adapted from Purtilo DT, Purtilo RB: A survey of human diseases, ed 2, Boston, 1989, Little, Brown & Co, Inc.

Treatment Principles

The medical management of a patient with cancer includes surgery, radiation therapy, chemotherapy, and bone marrow transplant. These interventions are responsible for an enhanced survival rate. Physical therapists and physical therapist assistants have become more involved with these patients as their remission periods have increased. However, physical therapy intervention continues to focus on patients who are more severely involved. A study conducted in 1991 of all the members of the Oncology Section of the APTA revealed that 69 percent of the respondents were involved with patients who had cancer in Stage III or IV, while 31 percent of the respondents had patients with cancer in Stage I or II.[13] The most common diagnoses, in order of frequency were breast cancer, lung cancer, prostate cancer, hematological malignancies (e.g., leukemia), conditions related to AIDS, and cancers with metastases to the central nervous system. The most common reasons for the physical therapy referral were (in order) mobility training, strengthening exercises, pain management, range-of-motion exercises, and patient and family education.

Physical therapy intervention for a patient with cancer is usually coordinated with a team approach to care. This is a result of the widespread impact of the disease on the patient's body, mind, and family. Regarding the physical rehabilitation of the patient, four treatment principles have been described (Box 12-5).[2,3,7] The actual physical therapy techniques are no different from those for any individual with pain or decreased strength and/or range of motion, except that the extent of the dysfunctions is widespread and progressive. Each program must be unique to the needs of the patient. Special consideration must be given to post-operative complications such as swelling and decreased cardiopulmonary function.

Box 12-5

> ## Rehabilitation Goals for the Patient with Cancer*
>
> 1. Preventive Rehabilitation—techniques to reduce the severity of the antic-ipated disability, e.g., bed activities to maintain joint range of motion and cardiopulmonary status.
>
> 2. Restorative Rehabilitation—techniques to expedite the patient's return to his/her previous lifestyle, e.g., post-operative exercises to regain strength and range of motion.
>
> 3. Supportive Rehabilitation—techniques to keep the patient an active participant in establishing maximum functional independence, e.g., assistive devices for independent ambulation.
>
> 4. Palliative Rehabilitation—techniques to reduce the severity of the disease as it progresses and spreads, e.g., transfer activities out of bed to enhance the patient's environment.

*   From Dietz JH, editor: Rehabilitation oncology, Somerset, NJ, 1981, John Wiley and Sons.

The physical therapist and physical therapist assistant must also be sensitive to the psychosocial impact of the disease. The diagnosis itself is associated with negative outcomes such as pain, loneliness, and death.[14] The physical therapist (PT) and phys-ical therapist assistant (PTA) must respond to these perceptions by being supportive, yet honest. Family members will become involved with the emotional and physical impact of the disease. In order to avoid burnout, the PT and PTA should have their own support mechanisms to cope with the stress and frustrations of the disease. These may include routine team meetings with the mental health provider (social worker, psychologist).[7] By being honest and realistic with their own feelings, the PT and PTA will be more effective in their communication and interaction with the patient and family.

INDUSTRIAL REHABILITATION

Description

Industrial rehabilitation involves treatment and prevention programs for work-related injuries. The goals are to safely return the individual to work and increase produc-tivity.[11] This is a relatively new area for physical therapists and physical therapist assis-tants; however, it continues to expand as health care providers and employers seek effective methods to maintain and increase employee health and productivity. Both treatment and prevention programs include detailed evaluations (including job sites and activities), education, training, and exercises designed for specific work-related tasks. These areas will be presented in this section.

Functional Capacity Assessment

Industrial rehabilitation has had an impact on the evaluation and treatment components of health care that is focused on returning the individual safely to work. Following an injury and a traditional plan of care, a specific evaluation is performed to initiate an industrial rehabilitation program. This is the **functional capacity assessment** and may continue for several days.[19] (In this area of health care, which is developing rapidly, a functional assessment is also known as a functional capacity assessment, physical capacity evaluation, worker assessment, functional capacity evaluation, and work capacity evaluation.[11])

As described by Key, the functional capacity assessment consists of four components: (1) weighted capabilities, (2) tolerances, (3) participation level, and (4) postural examination.[11] The **weighted capabilities** component consists of an evaluation of the individual's ability to transfer materials of varying weights. **Tolerances** refers to the length of time an employee can safely perform an activity throughout the workday (e.g., can stand for one-hour periods for a total of four hours). These numbers must be carefully established to ensure the appropriate participation level of the individual. Different methods are available to set activity levels for high patient/client compliance. The final component, **postural examination,** is an analysis of the postural changes of the patient/client while performing the job activity in a simulated environment. At this stage, the therapist must not provide correction, otherwise the results of the evaluation will be faulty. The postural examination must reflect actual performance of the given activity.

Job Analysis

Following the functional capacity assessment which was conducted in a controlled environment, the therapist must go to the job site to conduct a similar assessment in the actual work environment. Two analyses are conducted here, one of the job task and another of the job site.[17] The **job task analysis** is quantitative in nature and includes measurements of weights, distances, repetitions, and cycle times. The **job site analysis** is qualitative in nature and includes descriptions of the work station (including materials and tools) and activities performed (including body positions and movements). Results of these analyses are integrated with the results from the functional capacity assessment to establish a treatment program.

Treatment Principles

Interventions for an individual with a work-related injury can be categorized into **work-conditioning programs** or **work-hardening programs** (Table 12-1).[16] In both programs, the goal is to return the individual to work. However, the former focuses more on the physical dysfunctions (e.g., strength, range of motion, and cardiovascular endurance) while the latter is broader in scope to include behavioral and vocational management (e.g., counseling). When the program is completed, a discharge evaluation is conducted to compare to the initial evaluation (functional capacity assessment). This provides an opportunity to determine the effectiveness of the program and the individual's level of ability in the work environment.

Table 12-1: Comparison of Work-Conditioning and Work-Hardening Programs*

Work-Conditioning Program	Work-Hardening Program
1. Addresses physical and functional needs.	1. Addresses physical, functional, behavioral, and vocational needs.
2. Single discipline (e.g., PT) approach.	2. Interdisciplinary approach.
3. Uses exercises and activities related to work.	3. Uses exercises and activities in real or simulated environment.
4. Provided in multi-hour sessions up to four hours/day, five days/week, for eight weeks.	4. Provided in multi-hour sessions between four and eight hours/day, five days/week, for up to eight weeks.

*   Adapted from Resource guide: industrial physical therapy, Alexandria, VA, 1992, American Physical Therapy Association.

Prevention

Recently, the business and health care industries have been collaborating to establish health promotion programs to prevent injury and disease and thereby reduce health care costs while increasing productivity. Physical therapists and physical therapist assistants are directly involved with these health promotion and disease prevention programs. These individuals may serve as consultants to establish programs or as health care providers to deliver services either on site or in a health-related facility.

Prevention programs generally include several components: (1) history questionnaire, (2) medical screening and evaluation, (3) consultation, (4) exercise performance, and (5) re-assessments.[10] The history questionnaire provides information about general health and related habits. A comprehensive medical and physical evaluation is necessary to establish a baseline and design a program. Consultation is provided individually or in a group to describe the results of the evaluation and compare them to norms. Exercise programs are designed based on evaluation results. They may be conducted at home, at work, or at a health-related facility. Re-assessments are done periodically to ensure program effectiveness and serve as a motivating factor.

SUMMARY

Selected topics were presented in this chapter to describe a variety of physical therapy practice areas which did not necessarily apply to one of the previous chapters. These topics also serve to demonstrate the breadth of the profession. The physical therapy management of the patient with AIDS was described with special attention to the HIV-infected child and ethical responsibility to render treatment. Aquatic physical therapy, as distinguished from hydrotherapy, was presented as a treatment which has gained recent interest, but it has existed since the origins of physical therapy in the United States. The pathophysiology of burns was presented to demonstrate the severity of this injury, followed by physical therapy interventions to restore function. The physical therapy management of the patient with cancer was described as a comprehensive physical program with sensitivities to the psychosocial impact of the disease. In the final topic, industrial rehabilitation, management of work-related injuries was described with the goal of returning the individual to work in a safe, productive environment. Prevention programs were included in this topic to indicate that physical therapists and physical therapist assistants are directly involved in health promotion and disease prevention programs.

References

1. APTA Aquatic Physical Therapy Section Statement of Purposes, Rationale, and Goals, Alexandria, VA, 1992, American Physical Therapy Association.

2. Dietz JH, editor: Rehabilitation oncology, Somerset, NJ, 1981, John Wiley and Sons.

3. Etherington M: Physical therapy management of the cancer patient, Clin Manage in Phys Ther 7(3):12-15, 1987.

4. Galantino ML: An overview of the AIDS patient, Clin Manage in Phys Ther 7(2):12-13, 1987.

5. Galantino ML, Levy JK: HIV-infection: neurological implications for rehabilitation, Clin Manage in Phys Ther 8(1):6-13, 1988.

6. Giuliani CA, Perry GA: Factors to consider in the rehabilitation aspects of burn care, Phys Ther 65(5):619-623, 1985.

7. Hamburgh, RR: Principles of cancer treatment, Clin Manage in Phys Ther 12(4):37-41, 1992.

8. Haralson KM: Therapeutic pool programs, Clin Manage in Phys Ther 5(2):10-13, 1985.

9. Harris-Copp M: The HIV-infected child, Clin Manage in Phys Ther 8(1):16-19, 1988.

10. Huhn RH, Volski RV: Primary prevention programs for business and industry, Phys Ther 65(12):1840-1844, 1985.

11. Key GL: Industrial physical therapy. In Gould JA III, editor: Orthopaedic and sports physical therapy, ed 2, St. Louis, 1990, CV Mosby Company.

12. Morris DM, Irion JM, Charness AL: Agnatic physical therapy as a procedure. In Cirullo JA, editor: Aquatic physical therapy. Orthopaedic Physical Therapy Clinics of North America 3(2), Philadelphia, 1994, WB Saunders Co.

13. Pfalzer L, Walter J: Facts and fiction: cancer in the 1900s, Clin Manage in Phys Ther 12(4):26-31, 1992.

14. Position on infectious diseases, HOD 06-89-39-84, Alexandria, VA, 1989, American Physical Therapy Association.

15. Purtilo DT, Purtilo RB: A survey of human diseases, ed 2, Boston, 1989, Little, Brown & Co.

16. Resource Guide: industrial physical therapy, Alexandria, VA, 1992, American Physical Therapy Association.

17. Sim J, Purtillo RB: An ethical analysis of physical therapists' duty to treat persons who have AIDS: homosexual patients as a test case, Phys Ther 71(9):650-655, 1991.

18. Wright PC: Fundamentals of acute burn care and physical therapy management, Phys Ther 64(8):1217-1231, 1984.

19. Wynn KE: A continuum of care to treat the injured worker, PT-Magazine of Phys Ther 2(1):52-54, 1994.

20. Wynn KE: Lily ponds, warm springs, and fortunate accidents, PT-Magazine of Phys Ther 2(12):44-45, 1994.

Suggested Reading

Key G: Industrial Therapy, St. Louis, MO, 1995, Mosby-Year Book. This comprehensive text covers industrial therapy in the contemporary workplace, including injury prevention, returning the worker to productivity, and the management of industrial therapy.

Review Questions

1. Prepare a report on universal precautions procedures. Add examples of their application in a physical therapy setting.

2. Without looking at your book, list as many contraindications to aquatic therapy as you can.

3. Use library sources to research and report briefly on the kinds of damage done by each of the three causative agents of burns: thermal, electrical, or chemical.

4. Your text talks about using specific "resting positions" for burn patients. Predict and then research to discover the purposes/benefits of such positions. Were your predictions right?

5. Imagine you are a PT or a PTA serving the oncology patients in a large hospital. Describe the most important concerns and aspects of your specialized area of practice.

6. Develop two specific cases of intervention programs in response to a work-related injury to differentiate between work-conditioning and work-hardening programs.

Glossary

accessory motion: Ability of the joint surfaces to glide, roll, and spin on each other.

acquired immunodeficiency syndrome (AIDS): Diagnosis based on both a positive test for the human immunodeficiency virus (HIV) and the presence of an opportunistic infection or malignancy.

active range of motion (AROM): Ability of the patient to voluntarily move a limb through an arc of movement.

active-assisted ROM: Joint movement in which the patient may be assisted either manually or mechanically through an arc of movement.

active-free ROM: Joint movement in which the patient does not receive any support or resistance through an arc of movement.

active-resisted exercise: Joint movement in which an external force resists the movement.

adaptive equipment/assistive device: Any device that enables an individual to accomplish a functional task with increased ease or independence.

aerobics training: Exercise program that uses oxygen as major energy source.

Affiliate Assembly: Component of the APTA that represents and is comprised of PTAs.

Affiliate Special Interest Group: Past component of the APTA; precursor to Affiliate Assembly.

akinesia: A poverty of movements.

alliance: Collaboration of several health care facilities and practices.

ambulatory center: Any facility in which health care is provided on an outpatient basis; the patient is able to walk into the facility, receive care, and walk out of the facility the same day.

American Board of Physical Therapy Specialties: Unit created by the House of Delegates to provide a formal mechanism for recognizing physical therapists with advanced knowledge, skills, and experience in a special area of practice.

American Physical Therapy Association (APTA): National organization that represents physical therapists in the U.S.A.

American Physiotherapy Association (APA): Organization (formerly called American Women's Physical Therapeutic Association) responsible for maintaining high standard and educational programs for physiotherapists. Precursor to APTA.

American Women's Physical Therapeutic Association: First national organization representing "physical therapeutics." Established in 1921 to maintain high standards and provide a mechanism to share information.

amyotrophic lateral sclerosis (ALS): Also known as "Lou Gehrig's disease"; rapidly progressive neurological disorder associated with a degeneration of the motor nerve cells.

angina: Condition in which chest pain occurs from ischemia.

angiography: Injecting radiopaque material into the blood vessels to better visualize and identify problems such as occlusion (blockage) of blood vessels, aneurysms, and vascular malformations.

angioplasty: The process of mechanically dilating a blood vessel.

annual conference: Yearly (June) meeting of the APTA, held in accordance with the Bylaws, and usually including an extensive program of presentations and activities.

aquatic physical therapy: Therapeutic use of water for rehabilitation or prevention.

arteriosclerosis: Hardening of the arteries.

assembly: Component of APTA whose purpose is to provide a means by which members of the same class may meet, confer, and promote the interest of the respective membership class.

assessment: Measurement or assigned value by which physical therapists make a clinical judgment.

assessment process: In pediatric physical therapy, close monitoring, evaluation and, if indicated, initiation of treatment.

Bad Ragaz method: Aquatic therapy technique using proprioceptive neuromuscular facilitation techniques while the patient is suspended by rings in the water environment.

biological dressings: Homografts and heterografts.

blood gas analysis: Assessment of blood (usually arterial) to determine the concentration of oxygen and carbon dioxide.

Board of Directors (BOD): APTA unit consisting of six APTA officers and nine directors, whose duty is to carry out the mandates and policies established by the HOD.

bradykinesia: Slowness of movements.

Brunnstrom's approach: Neurological technique based on natural sequence of recovery following stroke.

bursitis: Inflammation of bursae, fluid-filled sacs located throughout the body that serve to decrease the friction between two structures.

cancer: A variety of diseases, all of which are characterized by uncontrolled growth and spread of abnormal cells.

cardiac catheterization: Passing a catheter (a flexible tube) into an artery in the arm or leg, then along the artery reaching the heart to measure pressure, inject dye, or take a sample.

cardiac muscle dysfunction: Various pathologies associated with heart failure.

cardiac pacemaker: Electronic device that produces a pulse which controls heart depolarization.

career ladder: Employer's structure, creating levels within a specific field or position to enable promotion of employees in that category.

cerebral palsy (CP): Group of conditions caused by a non-progressive lesion on the brain. Most often CP occurs during gestation (before birth), at birth, or immediately after birth, due to an interruption of oxygen to the brain of the fetus or newborn.

chapter: Organizational unit of the APTA which is defined by specific legally constituted boundaries such as a state, territory, or commonwealth of the United States or the District of Columbia. Membership is automatic, based on location of residence, employment, education, or greatest active participation.

chronic obstructive pulmonary disease (COPD): Group of disorders that produce certain specific physical symptoms, including chronic productive cough, excessive mucus production, changes in the sound produced when air passes through the bronchial tubes, and shortness of breath (dyspnea).

closed chain exercises or kinetic chain exercises: Those exercises incorporating several muscle groups through the use of several joints with the end segment fixed.

clubfoot: Disorder in which the foot is turned inward and slanted upward.

Code of Ethics: Principles set forth for the physical therapy profession by the APTA for maintaining and promoting ethical practice.

Combined Sections Meeting: Meeting in early February of APTA sections' members to provide an opportunity for sharing information.

Commission on Accreditation in Physical Therapy Education (CAPTE): Unit responsible for evaluating and accrediting professional (entry-level) physical therapy and physical therapist assistant educational programs.

common law: Law created by court decision rather than by legislative action.

computerized axial tomography (CAT scan): Computer synthesis of x-rays transmitted through a specific plane of the body.

conducting airways: Passageways and tubes that allow air to pass into or out of the lungs.

conductive education: Based on motor learning concepts in which disability is a result of the interaction between the child and the environment. One individual (a conductor) works with the child as an active learner by assisting her or him with completion of all daily activities while the child repeats rhythmic, verbal phrases describing her/his actions.

congenital dislocation of the hip (CDH): Dislocation resulting from the abnormal development of some of the structures surrounding the hip joint, allowing the head of the femur (thigh bone) to move in and out of the hip socket. Cause is unknown.

congestive heart failure (CHF): Condition in which the heart muscle is compromised to the point that it cannot move blood volume effectively.

Continuous Quality Improvement / Total Quality Management (CQI/TQM): Method of examining and improving processes using data management tools.

continuum of disablement: Attempt by the World Health Organization (WHO) to distinguish varying levels of disability/impairment and their specific impact on the individual.

coronary artery bypass grafting (CABG): Grafting (attaching) a small artery or a leg vein to a point beyond the blockage or plaque. This "bypasses" the blockage, establishing blood flow to the heart.

coronary heart disease (CHD): Arteriosclerosis, or a hardening of the arteries, affecting the coronary vessels.

critical pathways: Guideline for patient hospital care using "milestones" to monitor progress; based on consensus, including only those aspects of care provided to affect patient outcomes.

cross-training: Training health professionals in treatment skills from a variety of professions to provide a multi-disiplinary team in a patient-focused care (PFC) model.

cryotherapy: Application of cold agents causing a decrease in blood flow and decreased metabolism, which result in a decrease in swelling and pain.

cystic fibrosis (CF): Most common inherited chronic pulmonary disease among Caucasian children, characterized by the production of thick mucus with progressive lung damage.

deep heat modalities: Physical agents producing similar physiological effects to superficial heat agents, but affecting a greater depth of tissues. Includes ultrasound and short wave diathermy.

developmental delay (DD): Failure to attain predictable movement patterns or behaviors associated with children of a similar chronological age.

diagnosis: Final interpretation of findings based on examinations; in physical therapy this must be made in accordance with a policy adopted by the APTA House of Delegates.

direct access: Availability of the physical therapist to anyone seeking those services without stipulation of a referral by another health care provider.

disability: Manifestation of an impairment.

district: Most local organizational unit in the structure of the APTA. Membership is automatic and may be based on location of residence or employment, as provided in the bylaws of the APTA.

Division of Special Hospitals and Physical Reconstruction: Organization created in 1917 to train and manage aides (exclusively women) who would provide physical reconstruction to persons injured in war.

Down syndrome: Congenital developmental disability caused by a defect of the 21st chromosome; sometimes called Trisomy 21.

Duchenne muscular dystrophy (DMD): Progressive pelvic muscle weakness and wasting in the male child, combined with enlarged, yet weak, thigh muscles and tight heel cords.

dynamic balance: Balance maintained with the body in motion.

dynamic contraction: Muscular contraction performed through a full range of motion.

dysfunction: Any functional disability.

dyspnea: Shortness of breath.

echocardiography: Use of high frequency ultrasound to assess the size of the heart chambers, the thickness of the chamber's walls, and the motion of the chamber walls and heart valves.

eclectic approach: Combination of therapeutic approaches used by the physical therapist and thought to be useful for treatment of a given client.

electrical stimulation: Application of electricity at specified locations to stimulate nerves, muscles, and other soft tissues to reduce pain and swelling, to increase strength and range of motion, and to facilitate wound healing.

electrocardiography (ECG): Use of electrodes placed on the anterior chest wall to record depolarization or contraction of the heart muscle; assesses the heart's rate and rhythm.

electroencephalography (EEG): Recording of the electrical potential/activity in the brain by placing electrodes on the scalp.

electromyography (EMG): Recording the electrical activity in the muscle during a state of rest and during voluntary contraction.

embolus: Clot formed by a substance detached from elsewhere.

encroachment: Situation occurring in health care, in which one health care provider performs the skills and techniques of another health care provider.

evaluation: Process by which physical therapists make a clinical judgment based on an examination.

examination: Test used to obtain a measurement.

exercise stress testing: Noninvasive method of determining how the cardiovascular and pulmonary systems respond to controlled increases in activity; most frequently used to diagnose suspected or established cardiovascular disease.

expiration: Breathing out.

expressive aphasia: Impaired ability to express oneself.

family assessment: Family interview, survey, or other format generated to gain the family's insights regarding a patient—especially a child; includes family history, relationships, concerns, needs, and resources.

fetal alcohol syndrome (FAS): Most severe condition in a continuum of alcohol-induced disabilities related to high levels of maternal alcohol consumption during pregnancy.

first-degree burns: Burn resulting in a sunburn-like effect.

flexibility: Ability to move a limb segment through a range of motion.

flexibility exercise: Exercise used to change the length and elasticity of soft tissue, such as muscle, over time, using stress; usually for postural or ROM enhancement.

fluidotherapy: Use of a self-contained unit filled with sawdust-type particles heated to the desired temperature and circulated by air pressure around the involved body part.

form: Documentation method using a standard format.

frail elderly: People over 65 with conditions which significantly impair their daily function.

full-thickness burn: Burn that includes all the dermis; same as third-degree burn.

functional capacity assessment: Specific evaluation, performed following an injury and a traditional plan of care to initiate an industrial rehabilitation program.

functional exercises: Exercises that mimic functional movements and activities. Functional movements incorporate strength, flexibility, balance, and coordination.

functional reach test: Specific balance test that can predict the likelihood of falling.

gatekeeper: Health care provider who provides a consumer access into the health care system. Historically, this has been the primary care physician.

goals: Measurable, functional objectives that are linked to a problem identified in a patient evaluation.

goniometer: Instrument used to measure and document ROM.

goniometry: Methods to measure and document ROM.

Halliwick method: Aquatic therapy technique using a preswim stroke instruction and musculoskeletal rehabilitation.

handicap: Influence of social/environmental factors upon a disability.

health maintenance organization (HMO): Center which provides all health care services needed under one roof.

heart failure: A decrease in the pumping capability of the heart muscle.

heterografts: Tissue transferred between different species.

homografts: Tissue transferred between same species.

hot packs: Pouches filled with silica gel and soaked in thermostatically controlled water.

House of Delegates (HOD): Highest policy-making body of the APTA created in 1944.

hydrotherapy: Use of the therapeutic effects of water by immersing the body part or entire body into a tank of water.

hypermobile joint: Joint with excessive motion.

hypertonia: High tone.

hypomobile joint: Joint with less motion than is considered functional.

hypotonia: Low tone.

impairment: Level of disablement that *directly* affects the individual, particularly physically.

individualized education plan (IEP): Model using collaboration of therapists, family, educators, and other health team members to provide direct intervention in the classroom setting.

individualized family services plan (IFSP): Detailed total plan of care for the child in the context of the family unit.

informed consent: Client-granted permission to treat, required in accordance with the Standards of Practice approved by the APTA. Obtained by the physical therapist before rendering physical therapy.

infrared: Use of infrared radiation to warm the superficial tissue and create a general feeling of relaxation and pain relief.

inspiration: Contraction of the muscles of respiration, resulting in an increase in the space contained within the thoracic cavity. This expansion causes the air pressure to drop inside the lungs resulting in air moving into the lungs.

ischemia: Insufficient oxygenation of tissues due to a blocked blood vessel.

isometric contraction: Muscular contraction involving no motion.

job site analysis: Qualitative assessment of the work station (including materials and tools) and activities performed (including body positions and movements).

job task analysis: Quantitative assessment of the work environment including measurements of weights, distances, repetitions, and cycle times.

joint mobilization: Techniques used when a patient's dysfunction is the result of joint stiffness or hypomobility (loss of motion); applies specific passive movements to a joint, either oscillatory (rapid, repeated movements) or sustained.

juvenile rheumatoid arthritis: One of the many rheumatic diseases characterized by an inflammation of the connective tissue which manifests as a painful inflamed joint (arthritis); begins in childhood.

law: Formal rule laid down, ordained or established by a governing body.

licensure: Regulation designed to provide standards for a given public service and to thereby protect the public from harm.

ligaments: Supporting structures at joints that serve to stabilize the joint and prevent excess movement.

lumbar puncture: Injection of hypodermic needle into lumbar subarachnoid space.

magnetic resonance image (MRI): Computer image produced by placing the body part in a magnetic field.

malpractice: Injuries or wrongful behavior which a provider inflicts on a patient or client; negligence is the specific term used to describe this act. This involves a duty, a breach of that duty, and damage to the individual's person or property.

managed care network: Group of health care providers that form a professional cooperative relationship for the purpose of referring individuals to health care providers within the network.

managed care setting: Arrangement in which the insurance company contracts with health care providers to provide health care to the consumers who subscribe to the insurance plan.

manual muscle testing (MMT): Test allowing the therapist to assign a specific grade to a muscle, based on whether the patient can hold the limb against gravity, how much manual resistance can be tolerated, and whether there is full range of motion at a joint.

massage: Systematic use of various manual strokes designed to produce certain physiological, mechanical, and psychological effects.

meningocele: Benign herniation of the meninges presenting as a soft tissue cyst or lump that surrounds a normal spinal cord resulting in no neurological deficits.

meningomyelocele: Open congenital spinal cord lesion with minimal to no skin protection containing the deeper nerve roots.

motor control: Ability to manipulate movement and non-movement of the body's musculoskeletal components.

motor learning: Body's mechanism for acquiring or learning voluntary motor control.

multiple sclerosis (MS): Disease in which patches of demyelination occur in the nervous system, leading to disturbances in conduction of messages along the nerves.

muscle endurance: Ability to produce and sustain tension over a prolonged period of time.

muscular strength: Maximal amount of tension an individual can produce in one repetition.

myocardial infarction: Heart attack; one of the coronary arteries suddenly becomes blocked by an embolus (clot).

myofascial release: Manual stretching of the layers of the body's fascia (connective tissue that surrounds muscle and other soft tissues in the body).

narrative: Form of documentation that allows maximum flexibility, but is completely unstructured.

National Foundation for Infantile Paralysis ("Foundation"): Foundation established in 1938 in response to repeated polio epidemics. Established to provide research, education, and patient services.

negligence: Specific term used to describe an act of malpractice (injury or wrongful behavior that a client sustains from a physical therapy provider). It must involve three components: (1) a duty, (2) breach of duty, and (3) damage to the individual's person or property.

nerve conduction velocity (NCV) studies: Recording the rate at which electrical signals are transmitted along peripheral nerves.

nerve entrapment: Pressure on a nerve.

neurodevelopmental treatment approach (NDT): Approach to both analyze and treat neurological disorders of posture and movement. Through the use of a motivating environment and a patient's active participation, manual facilitation and inhibition techniques are employed by the therapist to present the patient with a "normal" sensory experience, thereby encouraging facilitation of a more functional motor response.

non-compete clause: Contract between employer and employee which stipulates certain conditions of practice following termination of employment, usually identifying a minimum length of time and distance within which the former employee cannot establish a practice which will compete with the original employer.

normal developmental theory: Model asserting that therapy goals and objectives are designed to follow the progression of normal motor development. Assumes that children with central nervous system damage will acquire motor skills in a similar fashion to children with normally developing nervous systems.

objective examination: Quantitative or qualitative measurements that are taken by the physical therapist or by use of a mechanical device.

obstructive lung disease: Pathological abnormality in air flow through the bronchial tubes.

old-old: Those 85 years or older.

open chain exercises or joint isolation exercises: Those exercises in which the end limb segment is free.

orthopaedics: Field of physical therapy that focuses on function and dysfunction of an individual's musculoskeletal system.

osteoarthritis: Condition characterized by degeneration of cartilage as a result of many years of use. Hands, spine, knees, and hips are most commonly affected.

osteogenesis imperfecta (OI): Common and severe bone impairment of genetic origin. Affects the formation of collagen during bone development, resulting in frequent fractures during the fetal or newborn period.

osteoporosis: Decreased mineralization of the bones caused by a decreased production of new bone cells and an increased resorption of bone.

paraffin treatment: A mixture of melted paraffin wax and mineral oil maintained at a specific temperature; used to promote relaxation and pain relief effects and greater comfort during range-of-motion exercises.

paraplegia: Spinal cord damage and resultant loss of sensory or motor function affecting the lower trunk and legs.

Parkinson's disease: Progressive condition also referred to as paralysis agitans and idiopathic parkinsonism, characterized by a classic triad of symptoms.

partial-thickness burns: Burn in which the layer of dermis is still intact.

passive range of motion (PROM): Amount of movement at a joint that is obtained by the therapist moving the segment without assistance from the patient.

patient-focused care (PFC): Patient-care model in which all departments in a hospital are decentralized, and professional staff are assigned to work on multidisciplinary teams; usually involves cross-training of health care professionals.

perception: Ability to integrate various simultaneous sensory inputs and to respond appropriately.

physiatrist: Title given to physicians who specialize in physical medicine.

physical therapist: Professional who works to evaluate, treat, and/or prevent physical disability, movement dysfunction, and pain resulting from injury, disability, disease, or other health-related conditions.

physical therapist assistant (PTA): Health care provider who assists the PT in the provision of physical therapy and has graduated from an accredited physical therapist assistant associate degree program.

physical therapy: Assessment, evaluation, treatment, and prevention of physical disability, movement dysfunctions, and pain resulting from injury, disease, disability, or other health-related conditions.

physical therapy aide: Non-licensed worker who is specifically trained, on the job, under the direction of a physical therapist.

physician-owned physical therapy service (POPTS): Physical therapy services owned or invested in by a physician.

physiotherapist: Synonym for *physical therapist;* commonly used outside the U.S.

physiotherapy: Another term for physical therapy, commonly used outside the U.S.; used by the first national organization, American Women's Physical Therapeutic Association.

policy: Plan or course of action designed to influence and determine decisions. APTA further defines this as "a decision which obligates actions or subsequent decisions on similar matters."

"post-professional" education: Advanced education of a licensed physical therapist, either at the certificate, master's, or doctorate level.

postural examination: Analysis of the postural changes of the patient/client while performing a job activity in a simulated environment.

practice act: A state's official statement or document of definition and regulation of a specific profession, setting down guidelines for those practicing the profession within its jurisdiction.

preferred provider: Provider (i.e., physical therapist) in a managed care setting who has contracted with a specific insurance company to provide health care to the consumers who subscribe to the specified insurance plan.

prenatal cocaine exposure: Fetal exposure to cocaine in utero due to maternal cocaine use during pregnancy. Infants often present with clinical signs of exposure after birth including hyperirritability, poor feeding patterns, high respiratory and heart rates, increased tremulousness, and irregular sleeping patterns.

presbycusis: Decreased ability to perceive higher pitches and to distinguish between similar sounds.

profession: Career or means of employment demonstrating five characteristics: commitment to field, a representative organization, knowlege in a specific area, social service, and recognized autonomy.

"professional" physical therapy education: All academic programs that prepare students for *entry* into the field of physical therapy, regardless of the degree.

proprioception: One's awareness of position and movement.

proprioceptive neuromuscular facilitation (PNF): Technique used to enhance movement and motor control, emphasizing proprioceptive (joint and position sense) stimuli, but also using tactile, visual, and auditory stimuli.

proprioceptors: Receptors found in the skin and joints which respond to stimuli such as pressure, stretch, and position.

pulmonary function test: Assessment of the effectiveness of the respiratory musculature and the integrity of the airways and lung tissues to help classify lung disease pattern into obstructive or restrictive.

quadriplegia: Spinal cord damage resulting in loss of sensory or motor function affecting all limbs.

qualitative measurement: Measurement or evaluation performed by observing and describing patterns of movement and/or deformities.

quantitative measurement: Measurement or evaluation in which specific numbers or grades may be assigned.

range-of-motion (ROM) exercise: Exercise for mobility of a joint. Falls into two categories: active or passive. Active ROM exercise involves voluntary movement of a limb through an arc of movement; passive ROM exercise involves the *therapist* moving the limb without patient assistance.

receptive aphasia: Diminished ability to receive and interpret verbal or written communication.

Reconstruction Aides: Aides (exclusively women) responsible for providing physical reconstruction to persons injured in war. Forerunners of the profession and practice of physical therapy in the United States.

regulation: Administrative or departmental statement issued to carry out the intent of the law.

reimbursement: System of health care payment through health insurance obtained through an employer, private insurance, Medicare, or Medicaid.

resisted exercise: Form of active movement in which some form of resistance is provided to increase muscular strength and endurance.

resisted test: Test that allows the therapist to determine the general strength of a muscle group and assess whether any pain is produced with the muscle contraction.

respiration: Process of exchanging oxygen and carbon dioxide between the air we breathe and the cells of the body.

Respondeat Superior: Concept that places the service responsibility on the supervisor or employer.

restrictive lung disease: Pathological reduction of the volume of air in the lungs.

rheumatoid arthritis: Chronic inflammation of the joints, of unknown etiology.

rigidity: Disturbance of muscle tone; manifests as a resistance when the limbs are passively moved.

Rood's approach: Neurological treatment using a variety of sensory stimuli to influence motor behavior.

scoliosis: Lateral curvature of the spine; may be idiopathic (unknown origin), neuromuscular, or congenital (present at birth).

screening: Examination indicated when there is risk of a developmental delay or disability.

second-degree burn: Burn resulting in a blister.

section: National level of organizational unit of the APTA. Membership is voluntary.

sation: Ability to receive sensory input from within and outside the body and transmit it through the peripheral nerves and tracts in the spinal cord to the brain, where it is received and interpreted.

sensory integration (SI) theory: Technique based on the theory that poor integration and use of sensory input (feedback) prevents subsequent motor planning (output). Providing controlled vestibular and somatosensory experiences enables the child to integrate the sensory information to evoke a spontaneous, functional response.

short-wave diathermy: Use of electromagnetic energy to produce deep therapeutic heating effects.

SOAP note: Documentation format taken from the Problem-Oriented Medical Record System; its components are (1) Subjective (what patient/family member describes, (2) Objective (what the PT observes/measures), (3) Assessment (clinical judgment based on evaluation; includes goals), and (4) Plan (treatment plan).

soft tissue mobilizations: Variety of "hands-on" techniques designed to improve movement and decrease pain.

special interest groups: Groups existing at multiple levels of the APTA to enable members at all levels to further organize into smaller specialty areas.

spina bifida: Congenital incomplete closure of a vertebra.

spina bifida occulta: Congenital incomplete closure of a vertebra (separation of the spinous process) that is not associated with disability.

spinal muscular atrophy (SMA): Genetic disorder characterized by severe muscle weakness in infancy and progressive respiratory failure.

spirometer: Instrument measuring the various volumes and airflow rates, which are then compared to a normal scale.

sprain: Overstretching of a joint ligament accompanied by a tearing of the fibers, causing pain and instability of the joint.

standardized testing: Type of formal test in which the evaluation procedures remain the same when administered by different therapists and at variable test locations.

Standards of Ethical Conduct for the Physical Therapist Assistant: Principles set forth by the APTA for maintaining and promoting high standards of professional conduct among affiliate member physical therapist assistants.

Standards of Practice for Physical Therapy: APTA document that addresses the administration of services and plan of care, as well as the education, research, community, and ethical/legal responsibilities of the physical therapist.

static balance: Balance maintained while standing still.

static contraction: Muscular contraction involving no motion.

statute: Formal written enactment of any legislative body at any governmental level.

strain: Tearing of muscle fibers, caused by a sudden contraction of a muscle or excessive stretch to the muscle.

strength: Amount of force produced during a voluntary muscular contraction.

stroke or cerebrovascular accident (CVA): Neurological problem arising from disruption of blood flow in the brain.

Student Assembly: Officially recognized component of the APTA whose members are physical therapy and physical therapist assistant students; provides a forum in which PT/PTA students can better understand their roles.

subjective: Term referring to data obtained from the patient's feelings and perceptions.

subjective evaluation/examination: Interviewing the patient about the extent and nature of an injury; a qualitative measurement based on the patient's perception of the problem.

survivor: An individual diagnosed with cancer who has experienced a five-year or greater remission period. However, the National Coalition for Cancer Survivorship defines a survivor as "anyone who's received a cancer diagnosis, whether treatment is being received or has been completed."

target heart rate (THR): Appropriate heart rate to be maintained during the peak period in aerobic training; calculated as a percentage of the individual's maximum heart rate.

tendinitis: Inflammation of a tendon, a structure located at the ends of muscles and that attaches muscle to bone.

thermal agents: Agents used to modify the temperature of surrounding tissue, resulting in a change in the amount of blood flow to the injured area.

third-degree burn: Burn that includes all the dermis; same as full-thickness burn.

tolerance: Length of time an employee can safely perform an activity throughout the workday.

tone: Tension exerted and/or maintained by muscles at rest and during movement.

training zone: An individual's ideal range of minimum and maximum heart rates (see target heart rate) that must be achieved for that individual to produce an aerobic training effect.

treatment plan: Selection of treatment activities related to established goals, based on patient diagnosis; it should include frequency and duration.

tremor: Alternating contractions of opposing muscle groups.

ultrasound: Therapeutic application of high frequency sound waves that penetrate through tissue and cause an increase in the tissue temperature to promote healing and reduce pain.

ventilation: Process of inspiration and expiration; results in an exchange of oxygen and carbon dioxide between the air found in the lungs and the pulmonary circulation.

Watsu: Aquatic therapy technique using application of Shiatsu in the water for relaxation.

weighted capability: Evaluation of the individual's ability to transfer materials of varying weights.

well elderly: People 65 years and over who are not experiencing physical limitations or who have age-related changes that are not significant enough to affect function.

whirlpool: Tank of water used in hydrotherapy for immersing a body part or the entire body.

work-conditioning programs: Interventions for an individual with a work-related injury, focusing mostly on physical dysfunctions (e.g., strength, range of motion, and cardiovascular endurance).

work-hardening programs: Interventions for an individual with a work-related injury, broad in scope to include behavioral and vocational management (e.g., counseling) as well as physical dysfunction.

young-old: Those in the 65–84 age range.

Index